HADASSAH
for the Health
of the People

I0628231

Prof. Shifra Shvarts
Dr. Zipora Shehory-Rubin

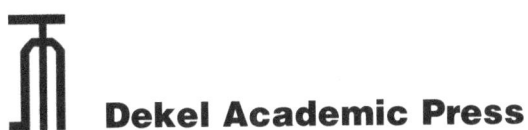

Dekel Academic Press

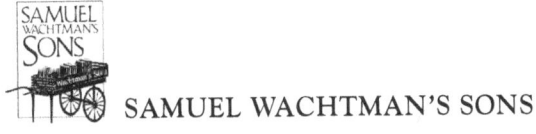

SAMUEL WACHTMAN'S SONS

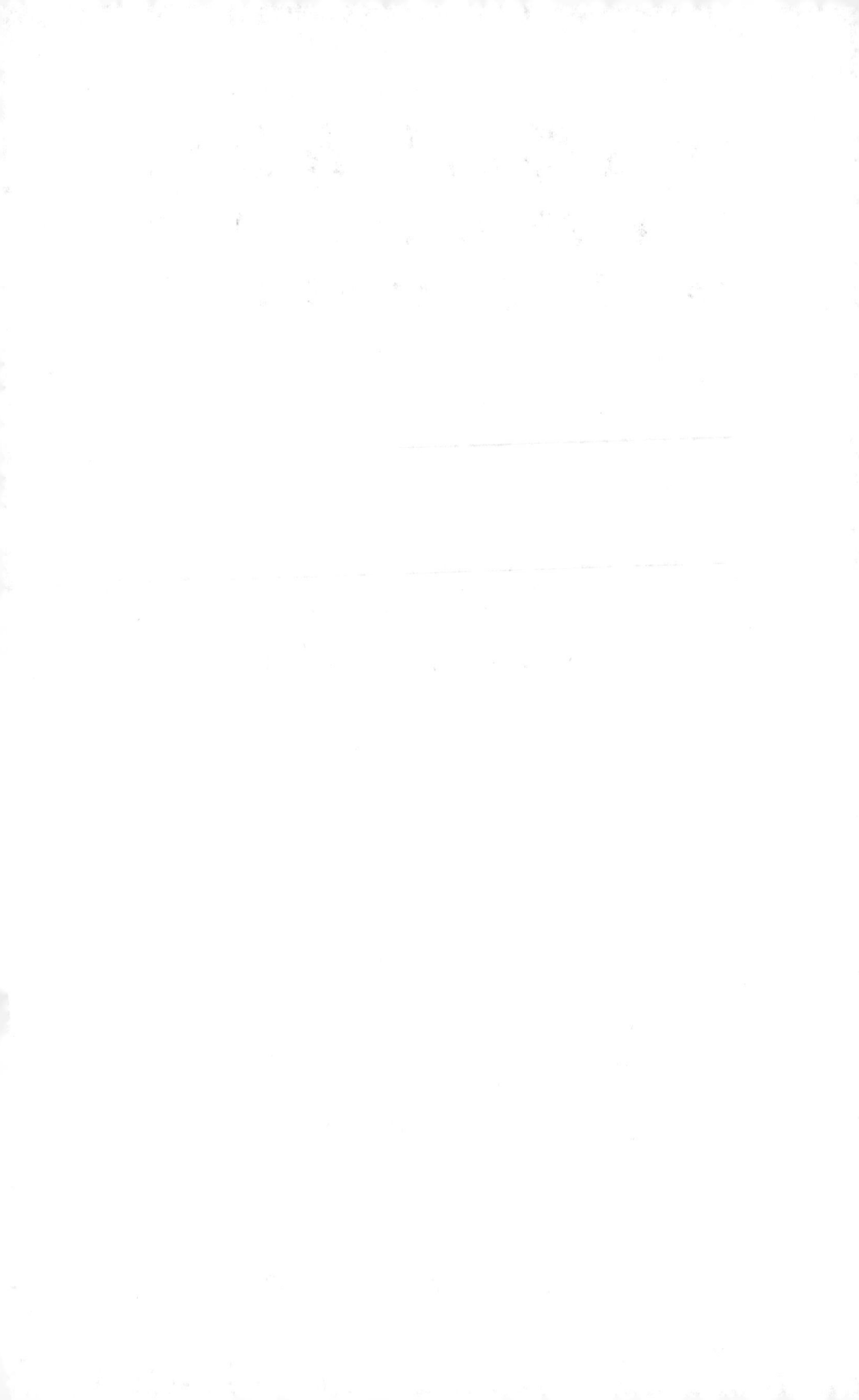

HADASSAH
for the Health
of the People

The Health Education Mission of Hadassah:
The American Zionist Women in the Holy Land

Prof. Shifra Shvarts
Dr. Zipora Shehory-Rubin

PHOTOGRAPHS BY COURTESY OF
Prof. Yoel Donchin,
Hadassah Historical Photograph Collection

WITH

Nancy Falchuk,
National President of Hadassah,
"Hadassah: 100 Years of Building Israel"

Prof. Shlomo Mor Yosef,
"Hadassah Then and Now"

George A. Silver, M.D.
Introduction

HADASSAH for the Health of the People
Prof. Shifra Shvarts & Dr. Zipora Shehory-Rubin
Copyright © 2012

Dekel Academic Press
www.dekelpublishing.com
ISBN 978-965-7178-22-5

North American Rights by
Samuel Wachtman's Sons, Inc.
ISBN 978-1-888820-40-9

Cover design: Studio Zafrir
Language editing: Katie Roman
Proofs reading: Pnina Ophir

Historical photographs by courtesy of:
Donchin-Hadassah Collection
Hadassah Archives, N.Y.
Rothschild-Hadassah Archives, Jerusalem

Interior design and typesetting by:

For information contact:

Dekel Academic Press
P.O. Box 45094
Tel Aviv 61450, Israel
Tel: +972 3506-3235
Fax: +972 3506-7332
Email: info@dekelpublishing.com

Samuel Wachtman's Sons, Inc.
2460 Garden Road, Suite C
Monterey, CA 93940, U.S.A.
Tel: 831 649-0669
Fax: 831 649-8007
Email: samuelwachtman@gmail.com

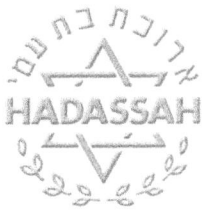

Acknowledgements

For both of us, as the authors of this work, the publication of this volume presents a pleasurable and long-awaited opportunity to thank all those who assisted us in our research and in the publication process.

To employees at the Hadassah Archives in New York City and the Central Zionist Archives in Jerusalem, for your interest in our research topic and your assistance in locating relevant documents; to Professor Shlomo Mor Yosef, director-general of the Hadassah Medical Federation for your invaluable support and generous assistance in making publication of the work possible; to Hadassah member, Andrea Kron from Los Alamos, NM, for her invaluable cartography of Hadassah Timeline and Hadassah institutions in Israel then and now; to Zvi Morik, Managing Director of Dekel Academic Press for the skillful and professional editing of the manuscript; to Katie Roman, our language editor and to DesignPeaks, our graphic editor, for your care and professionalism in overseeing the volume's final form and design; to our esteemed teacher and mentor, Professor Samuel Kottek, for reading the work and providing important insights that contributed greatly to the quality of the thesis; to Daniella Ashkenazy, who translated the original Hebrew manuscript into English, for the clarity of your translation and constructive comments and suggestions; to Judith Steiner-Freud for your unique prospective and the invaluable input you provided as a Hadassah nursing professional and as a scholar; to Dr. Nira Bartal for your assistance in elucidating the character of Hadassah nurses in Eretz Israel; to our fellow colleagues in the Israel Society for the History of Medicine and Science for the information of relevance to us that so many of you graciously shared with us;

and last but not least, to our families – the Shvartses and Rubins – for your unstinting encouragement, assistance and patience.

To all of you – our heartfelt thanks and gratitude.

The authors, July 2012
Ben Gurion University & Kaye Academic College of Education
Be'er Sheva, Israel

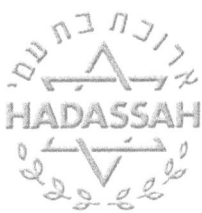

Table of Contents

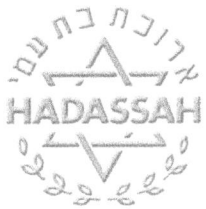

Dedicated to Prof. Samuel Kottek

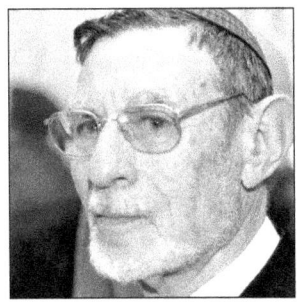

This book is dedicated to the life and work of Professor Samuel Kottek, a pediatrician at the Hebrew University-Hadassah School of Medicine, chairperson and scientific leader of the Israel Association for the History of Medicine and Science during the past 20 years.

In the course of three decades, Professor Samuel Kottek mentored an entire generation of medical historians whose scholarship focuses on the history of Jewish medicine. Professor Kottek is not only held in the highest esteem by his students as a teacher; he is venerated as an outstanding scholar, whose works on the unique facets of Jewish medicine during the Second Temple period are distinguished not only by their contribution to human knowledge but also by the author's strict impartiality and devotion to the truth, serving as a benchmark for those who have followed him. Professor Kottek's pioneering scholarship paved the way for other researchers to follow in his footsteps in the study of the uniqueness of Jewish medicine in *Eretz-Israel* and other Jewish communities following the destruction of the Second Temple and during the early Middle Ages.

His own seminal works continue to be an invaluable asset for all scholars of the history of Jewish medicine.

All of his published works are founded on thorough, in-depth investigation of archival material in order to extract the ideas, the prevailing moods and first and foremost the medical knowledge underlying the work of Jewish physicians during these periods – with special emphasis on the reciprocal impact of Jewish religious commandments and tradition, and medical practice and medical ethics on one another, and the relationship between medical theory that was current in the ancient world such as that of Hippocrates, and that held by Jewish physicians and Jewish medicine at the time.

Professor Kottek was born in Strasbourg in 1931 and graduated with honors from the University of Strasbourg School of Medicine in 1959. Upon graduation, he served in the Medical Corps of French forces in Algeria and in 1963 began his specialization in pediatrics. He studied the history of medicine under the late Professor Yehoshua Lebowitz, founder of the Israel Association for the History of Medicine and Science. In 1975 he immigrated to Israel and became a faculty member at the Hebrew University and in 1984 was appointed a professorship. In the course of his career, Professor Kottek served as a guest professor at leading institutions in the history of medicine, including Johns Hopkins in Baltimore, and the Wellcome Institute in London. For many years he served as a member of the board of the International Organization of the History of Medicine, and in the course of his academic career published more than 180 papers and four books. His scholarship was honored twice with the Muntner Price for the History of Medicine (1979, 1997), and the Einhorn Prize for Research in Hebrew Medical Language and Literature (1989). Although he retired in 2000, Professor Kottek continues his research in the history of medicine as professor emeritus at the Hebrew University in Jerusalem.

The book is a welcome addition to the literature that commemorates and celebrates over 30 year of scholarship that have gained Professor Kottek prominence as one of the leading researchers of the history of Jewish medicine in Israel and the Diaspora.

The authors

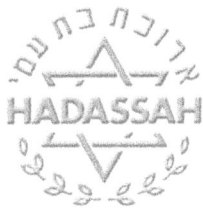

Hadassah: 100 Years of Building Israel
by Nancy Falchuk

Hadassah is a household name in Israel. The Hadassah Medical Center in Jerusalem is the pacesetter in Israeli medical treatment and research. The schools of medicine, dentistry and nursing that Hadassah operates with the Hebrew University are the bedrock of the nation's medical education system. Aside from the hundreds of thousands of Israelis who were born in or have been treated at one of Hadassah's hospitals, there are many more who have been treated by medical professionals trained at one of Hadassah's institutions of higher learning.

Less known by the Israeli public — especially the younger generations — is the story of how Hadassah's institutions came to occupy such a central position in Israeli life. In this volume, Shifra Shvarts and Zipora Shehory-Rubin tell the story of Hadassah in its formative years, during the British Mandate. In the three decades between the British conquest of Ottoman Palestine and the independence of modern Israel, Hadassah built a network of more than 130 hospitals, clinics, dispensaries and infant-welfare stations. That network was the medical and public health infrastructure of the future Jewish state.

Hadassah also built a substantial part of the emerging nation's educational foundation. In addition to the nursing school (founded during the Mandate period) and the medical and dental schools (opened in the first years after independence) Hadassah opened Youth Aliyah schools and villages to shelter and educate refugee children from Nazi-occupied Europe, and vocational schools that eventually evolved into today's Hadassah College Jerusalem.

But perhaps the least known part of the Hadassah story in Israel concerns the women behind the institutions. Hadassah, the Women's Zionist Organization of America, was founded in 1912, and those responsible for these key foundations of the Jewish state were nothing less than Hadassah's "Greatest Generation."

How did a women's organization in America come to play such a pivotal role in building a nation 10,000 kilometers away? The answer to this question highlights the dedication of Jewish women who came together to empower one another and also to work for a goal larger than themselves.

The Zionist idea of rebuilding the Jewish homeland found a ready audience in the distressed Jewish communities of Europe, but the success of Zionism in America was not pre-ordained. Most of America's Jewish population at the beginning of the twentieth century consisted of new immigrants whose idea of the Promised Land focused on the nation they or their parents had so recently chosen, not on the Middle East. Even those who were inclined to action had a long list of "isms" to choose from — socialism, unionism, capitalism, materialism, to name just a few.

Critical to Zionism's success in America was the development of Hadassah, especially the work of the organization's founder, Henrietta Szold. In 1909, at the age of 49, Szold visited Palestine and was horrified by the dismal public health conditions. In 1912, she transformed her women's study circle into Hadassah, with the idea of devoting members' energies to what she termed "practical Zionism." Ten months later, in January 1913, Hadassah dispatched two American nurses to Jerusalem to begin the organization's transformative medical mission.

All of this may sound straightforward in hindsight, but it is difficult to grasp today not only the medical challenges of the time but also the handicaps of those pioneers who set out to change the world. Hadassah was founded before women in America had the right to vote. Hadassah's Greatest Generation was a gathering of women in a men's world.

When they began, there was little room for them in the larger Zionist movement, so they carved out their own space. While other organizations engaged in debate and politics, Hadassah was determined to build. Few of those women had university educations. Few worked outside the home. They had no Blackberrys and no Internet. They worked to build a nation on the other side of the world that most of them would never see.

The first acknowledgment of Hadassah's success and expertise came early. After the privation of World War I, public health conditions in Palestine were even worse than what Henrietta Szold had witnessed just a few years before. When the Zionist Organization of America — at the request of the World Zionist Organization — moved to set up a large-scale medical mission to Palestine, it turned to Hadassah to spearhead the effort. That modest mission of two nurses on the eve of the war had given Hadassah something that existed nowhere else in the Zionist movement —experience in medical mobilization.

During the 1930s, as much of the world struggled through the Great Depression, Hadassah's development went into overdrive. Bolstered by a growing membership, the women of Hadassah crowned their healthcare network by building a flagship hospital on Mount Scopus. It was also during the 1930s that Henrietta Szold, by then living in Jerusalem, accepted responsibility for Youth Aliyah and Hadassah began sponsoring the Zionist youth movement Young Judaea. The organization emerged from the Depression stronger and more influential than ever.

The women of Hadassah's founding generation not only possessed boundless energy, they also made wise choices. They were smart enough to see what a nascent state needed to grow and what Jewish women in America needed to feel connected with the emerging nation. They were smart enough, and caring enough, to see that Zionism and Jewish values could only be served if the new medical institutions treated everyone equally, regardless of religion or ethnicity. They were smart enough to understand that a new nation couldn't keep importing expertise, but had to have its own educational foundation.

It is a Jewish characteristic to keep one eye on the future and one eye on the past, always balancing progress and innovation with tradition. This trait certainly describes Hadassah, striving to keep its institutions on the forward frontier of healing and learning and also strengthening the bonds of history and peoplehood that connect Israel with the Diaspora.

So it should not come as a surprise that in many ways Hadassah continues to do in the twenty-first century what it did during the years of the British Mandate — connecting hundreds of thousands of Jewish women to the land and people of Israel in practical ways.

The mission that began with two nurses and built some of Israel's critical foundations during the British Mandate continues today. In Hadassah's second century, American Jewish women — joined now by Hadassah groups in more than 25 countries around the world — connect people to Israel through medicine, research and education.

The greatest success of Hadassah's founding generation was to shrink the distance between itself and the Yishuv in Palestine. Today, no Jewish organization rooted in the Diaspora is more fully integrated into Israeli life than Hadassah. At the same time, Hadassah, more than any other Diaspora organization, has made Israel an integral part of itself.

Nancy Falchuk
Former National President of Hadassah
April 2011

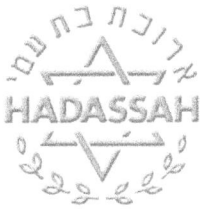

Hadassah Then and Now
by Prof. Shlomo Mor Yosef

In 1913, two American nurses arrived in Palestine to minister the health needs of the impoverished local residents. They were the vanguard of one of the greatest health initiatives of the twentieth century. They were the first undertaking of a fledging American Jewish women's organization called Hadassah, the Women's Zionist Organization of America (HWZOA). Those womens' extraordinary vision, unparalleled dedication and determination — and amazing accomplishments — have made Hadassah a watchword for healing for almost a century.

A trip to Palestine in 1909 was the turning point in the life of Henrietta Szold, Hadassah's founder — and in the future of health and welfare services in the country that became Israel. Shocked by her impressions of the dismal state of health care, she and her devoted followers set about to remedy the situation. Everything that followed transformed the landscape of Israel forever.

This book opens a window to those times and those that followed.

Branching out from the first Mother and Child Center in the Old City of Jerusalem, during the three decades of the British Mandate, Hadassah's ability to initiate and innovate set the standard for medicine in Israel. Establishing a network of clinics and hospitals throughout the country in the 1920s and 30s, they revolutionized the region — creating a public health infrastructure, introducing modern medical practices, promoting local care and global outreach, launching internationally acclaimed schools of medicine, nursing, dentistry and public health.

Turning away from the traditional European model, they imported standards from the United States. Their mission was to provide health care to all the people of the region in the most comprehensive manner.

From the beginning, the women of Hadassah focused on health and education. They concentrated their efforts in the community, considering it the most auspicious environment to develop and nurture their goals. And as they had from the start, they focused their efforts on children and young people.

Tipat Chalav, the well-baby clinics the women established, remain a major element of childcare in Israel today. Schools were not just a place for book learning. Hadassah saw them as centers for enriching and empowering children and educating them in healthy life styles. Concerned with nutrition, the women established hot breakfast and lunch programs; concerned with hygiene, they installed showers in the schools; concerned with physical health, they instituted medical checkups by doctors and nurses; concerned with mental health, they provided psychological services for children and their families. Based on social and educational principles, they established the first playgrounds in the country that were to play an essential role in the development of informal education.

This approach to encompass all aspects of people's health — physical and mental, psychological and social — was the hallmark of every area where HWZOA was involved. It has characterized the Hadassah Medical Organization ever since and in every situation.

Hadassah's activities laid the essential foundation for a modern system of health, medical, education and welfare services in the State of Israel. Hadassah wasn't alone. In pre-State Israel, it was an integral and inseparable part of a large group of Zionist organizations and institutions, whose relationships and power struggles were also an integral part of pre-State Israel. Yet, Hadassah's expertise was so renowned that in the days preceding the founding of the State, Hadassah was asked to assume responsibility for the nation's healthcare portfolio and with it, responsibility for organizing medical services in the country.

The revolution that Hadassah initiated in the early days of the last century continues until today. The two university hospitals in Jerusalem —

in Ein Kerem and on Mt. Scopus — continue to set a standard of excellence that others emulate. Hadassah's women's health centers and satellite services continue the Hadassah tradition of community involvement. Recently, Israel's health maintenance organizations changed their names — from sick funds to well funds — essentially validating Hadassah's belief that preventative medicine is as important as proper treatment.

Incorporating all medical and surgical sub-specialties, the Hadassah University Medical Center — home of the Hadassah Medical Organization — is a tertiary care referral facility, known for pioneering new medical techniques. A premier teaching hospital and research center, the Medical Center is equipped with the most sophisticated diagnostic, treatment and research equipment, which enables its world-renowned faculty to furnish the most modern medical care in an atmosphere that embraces excellence.

Hadassah treats some one million people each year in over 100 outpatient clinics and more than 70 departments and specialized units. A complete range of diagnostic laboratories as well as the most up-to-date imaging machines and other state-of-the-art equipment supports these clinical arms. Some departments are the only facilities of their kind in the Jerusalem area; others are unique in Israel, which has led the government to designate Hadassah as a National Center in a number of medical specialties. Professionals from all over the world come to learn from Hadassah's rich experience in patient care, teaching and research.

To solve medical mysteries, Hadassah created Centers of Excellence, a marriage of minds and systems. Their interdisciplinary team approach brings healing, teaching and research together in one place.

Research is a fundamental aspect of Hadassah's approach to comprehensive care. It offers solutions to present problems and paves the way for future treatments. Research is also the key to translational medicine, providing physicians with basic and clinical data to assist in patient treatment. Hadassah's physicians and scientists are actively engaged in a wide variety of extensive basic and clinical research projects, looking for new ways to treat current conditions. The cornerstone of Hadassah's philosophy is the interdependence between research and clinical services as the basis for quality care and the development of novel therapeutic approaches. For Hadassah, the physician-scientist is the most important player in the bench-to-bedside translational medicine approach.

The results of Hadassah's scientific investigations are reported in hundreds of academic papers published annually in leading professional journals, almost double the amount generated by any other Israeli hospital.

The Hadassah University Medical Center is known throughout the world for the outstanding education and clinical experience it provides in partnership with the Hebrew University at five schools of allied health professions. Located on the hospital campuses, they are hothouses of creativity for doctors, scientists and researchers in every medical field.

From its inception, Hadassah has extended its healing hand to all, without regard for race, religion, gender, political persuasion or ethnic origin. Our patients and staff are Jewish, Christian and Muslim — the religious and secular of each community. Hadassah offers its health services to people from far-off lands and from nearby regions, some from countries that don't recognize Israel, but who do understand the meaning of Hadassah.

Based on the belief that quality health care improves quality of life, Hadassah conducts a wide variety of training programs for medical personnel and students from the Palestinian Authority, Egypt and Jordan as well as numerous countries throughout the world. From Israel's earliest days, Hadassah has always extended a helping hand to other countries. From the rubble of earthquakes in Armenia, Turkey, Greece and Haiti to the battlefields of Cambodia, Rwanda and Kosovo; from terrorist bombings in Kenya and Argentina to refugee camps in Ethiopia, Hadassah's specialists have brought their expertise to nations in trouble and people in pain.

Today, nearly 100 years after the founding of their organization and more than six decades after the establishment of the State of Israel, the passions and principles that impelled Hadassah women to become involved during the days of the British Mandate remain unchanged.

From 1920 to 1933, Henrietta Szold divided her time between the United States and Palestine, directing the organization's activities at home and abroad. In 1933, she settled in Palestine and personally took on the responsibility of realizing the vision that changed her life — and the lives of countless others. Committing herself to her people and her land, her unbounded vision, indomitable spirit and practical Zionism created a culture of excellence that produced a system of health and welfare services for the benefit of all.

Hadassah's Zionist work has always been aimed at strengthening the Jewish State.

Just as you cannot describe the current Israeli health system without Hadassah, you cannot describe its beginnings without acknowledging the crucial role of the women of Hadassah.

Today, 100 years after the founding of their organization and more than six decades after the establishment of the State of Israel, the passions and principles that impelled Hadassah women to become involved during the days of the British Mandate remain unchanged. Hundreds of thousands of Hadassah members in the United States and thousands of Hadassah supporters in 20 countries across four continents remain steadfast in their historic commitment to health and education, as they will be far into the future. They act out of their strong feeling of shared destiny, deep devotion and enduring love for Hadassah – and through Hadassah, to Israel.

On Purim 2012, Hadassah will open the Sarah Wetsman Davidson Hospital Tower. This 19-story inpatient facility -- their centennial gift to the people of Israel – integrates Hadassah's deep dedication to healing with science's most sophisticated developing medical technologies.

Shlomo Mor Yosef
Hadassah Director General 2001-2011
July 2012

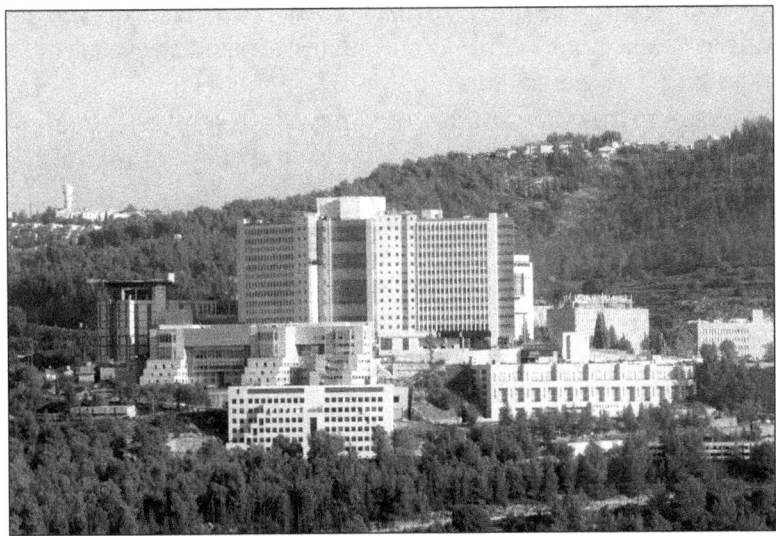

Hadassah University Medical Center, Jerusalem 2012.

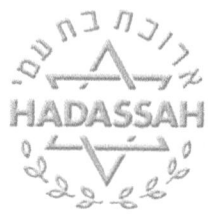

Introduction
by George A. Silver, M.D.

For the uninitiated, organizing a health care system afresh offers enticing possibilities.

One could avoid all errors of the existing system while designing in the improved programmatic details learned from one's experience. Also! Even as the medieval Hohenstaufen emperor learned in his efforts to determine what language humans would speak if they never heard the sound of a human voice, reality intervenes to prevent institution of social organization de novo. As we look at medical care structure worldwide, despite changes in form, certain basic problems remain. The Jews in Palestine in the early part of the twentieth century didn't even try to create a new design. They were anxious to develop a model medical care system that would meet their needs along the lines of the system they knew from their pre-Palestine lives. In a sense they saying they wanted something "as good as" and "like" the system in which they had grown up.

Later immigrants, however, who had had somewhat different experiences from different countries, introduced their own experiences into the pattern of medical care system organization, how it was paid and how it was controlled. The result was something like palimpsest — or a pentimento in artist's terminology — with each type of experience overlaid by another and visible remnants of each. At no time, it should be kept in mind, did the Jewish settlers ever see themselves as simply another

Middle Eastern tribe establishing another Middle Eastern state with a view to coping with the standard Middle Eastern problems in standard Middle Eastern ways. They accepted what existed, but aimed to transform the status quo into the futuristic vista of the Jewish state.

There had always been a thin layer of private practitioners around the cities, and this influenced the thinking of the planners. A little of the old Turkish practice remained and some British efforts to establish clinics were incorporated in settlers' thinking. Most of the immigrants had their views shaped by the nineteenth-century Bismarckian social insurance, emphasizing employment contributions for support and a capitated clinic style for delivery of services. The predominantly socialist politics of the settlers looked to trade union control as the key to management. For some, more government participation was desirable. When the Americans began to be active, through Hadassah, their ideas reflected what American social planners felt was desirable and necessary in the medical care system.

In the beginning of Hadassah activities, the emphasis was on nursing services, and, shortly, with the inheritance of the function of the American Zionist Medical Unit (as the Hadassah Medical Organization), promotion of public health and preventive services. There is no denying the tremendous boon this was to the Yishuv, in the light of the heavy load of communicable disease and tropical illnesses that the Jewish community faced. The eventual transfer of responsibilities for public health and preventive medicine from Hadassah to the Ministry of Health of the new state of Israel eased the pressures on the government for effective health services.

This historical review takes us from the organization of Hadassah medical involvement in Palestine in 1912 to the establishment of Jewish State of Israel. The early contribution, nursing, public health and preventive medicine were transformed, after the establishment of Israel, almost entirely into care responsibilities — the Hadassah Medical School and the Hadassah Hospital. With its strong focus on the American scene, Hadassah was powerfully committed to the ethos of American medicine while maintaining a strongly European texture. Almost all services continue to be covered in this way. Variations occur, even in European countries, such as the context of coverage — medications outside the hospital, for example. In most European countries, when a client earns above a certain income, full insurance coverage requires more premium payments. In European countries, state control is manifested through different agencies of government. In some countries, the Ministry of Social Affairs or a comparable agency is so charged. In others, the Ministry of Labor or Health takes responsibility. In any case, the Ministry of Health customarily takes responsibility for education, planning and setting medical practice standards. In Great Britain, instead of an insurance program, there is a full-scale guarantee of service and the medical care group (the National Health Service) is not simply guaranteed payment. Costs are met almost entirely out of general revenues, and the entire population is covered. Physicians and hospitals remain independent negotiators and are not government employees, but the system is under parliamentary control for budgeting and setting of standards.

Canada has developed a national medical care insurance program, in which the federal government provides about 50% of the amount spent by the provinces, and they in turn raise the rest through a variety of ways: a general state tax, joint employer–employee contributions, a special tax on state resources, or some combination of these. Again, physicians are private practitioners, not government employees, and hospitals are private institutions.

In all the national health programs, physicians negotiate their income with the governmental payment authority, while hospitals are generally reimbursed by way of direct budgeting procedures. Recent shifts in economic status and global changes in industrial practices have modified both state and private approaches to funding and administration of medical care services. However, historic forms have changed very little.

Eastern European countries redesigned their medical care system on the Soviet model after World War II, which directly controlled and operated their national health programs. Physicians were considered government employees and hospitals and clinics were government institutions. Bureaucratic and financial problems plagued these socialist-style health systems, but after the collapse of communism command economies declined in influence and previous centralized organizations for health care have undergone modification. However, their health systems have been cruelly buffeted by economic crises during the process of their shift to market economies.

In short, all the historic currents that influenced the organization and structure of medical care systems weighed on the Jewish community in Palestine and later on Israel. The early state model was closer to what the early immigrants recalled from their native lands. As successive experiences worked their influence, the original forms were modified and new forms were created to work with the old. Today's medical care in Israel reflects all these changes and the situation is still fluid. The role played by Hadassah in the organization and development of medical care and public health was critical and continues to exercise important influence through that early imprinting. Hadassah brought public health and preventive medicine into prominence as a governmental responsibility. It remains influential through medical education to create inventive and useful mechanisms for the improvement of medical care.

Israel is in an excellent position to test the value of certain organizational and administrative architecture for medical care service delivery. All European and the American models have demonstrated an inability to combine cost factors, quality of care and patient satisfaction into a national medical care program. And the struggle to define the roles of the government, medical centers and community organizations for modifying educational capability, defining biomedical research levels and satisfying medical care needs in economic and effective fashion has yet to be undertaken.

George A. Silver, M.D.
1914-2005

I would dare to believe that when an historian will come to write the chronicles of [the] Zionist settlement endeavor in Eretz Israel, he will have to say about Hadassah's project; It began as a simple form of assistance in wartime. It remained in the country as an important organization in peacetime. It became a vital part of the life blood of Eretz Israel, part and parcel of the rebirth Zionism strove to realize, and from beginning to end, remained faithful to its watchword: Arucat Bat-Ami.

Henrietta Szold

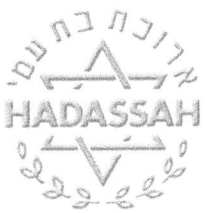

Chapter I

The Beginnings of Hadassah

In August 1898, under the leadership of Theodore Herzl, the Second Zionist Congress convened in Basel, Switzerland. Three hundred eighty-five delegates arrived, among them Richard Gottheil,[1] a professor of Semitic languages from Columbia University in New York. Professor Gottheil was accompanied by his wife, Emma. During their sojourn in Basel, Emma Gottheil met with Theodore Herzl, the father of modern Zionism — a movement designed to create a Jewish political and cultural entity in the ancient Jewish homeland. Herzl encouraged Emma Gottheil to organize American Jewish women on behalf of the Zionist cause.[2]

This meeting served as a catalyst and signaled the advent of a new period in the history of American Zionism. Emma Gottheil returned to the United States and established Jewish study groups comprised of Jewish women in their twenties. The groups focused on various Jewish issues and called themselves Daughters of Zion.

Other study groups sprang up in New York and Harlem. Most called themselves Daughters of Zion, but others adopted names of heroic Jewish women such as Deborah, Rebecca and Hadassah. This form of organization was common among women activists in social matters. Gottheil's study group was among the groups whose members — under the encouragement of Rabbi Judah-Leib Magnes,[3] rabbi of Temple Emanuel — later became leaders of American Zionist women. Among the women who joined Gottheil's group was Henrietta Szold, who became the group's leader. Thus was formed the nucleus of what would subsequently become the national organization of Zionist women.

On February 24, 1912, the founding groups of what was destined to become Hadassah convened with the purpose of establishing a pro-Zionist organization "to promote Jewish institutions and enterprises in Palestine and fostering Zionist ideals in America."[4]

Henrietta Szold — who had just returned from a visit to Eretz Israel — told the gathering about the arduous conditions prevailing in Jerusalem, Tiberias and Safed, particularly the dire state of hygiene, which, in her estimation, constituted the primary factor affecting the health of the Jewish community. She stressed the scope of the social-educational-health problem and underscored the need for an immediate and comprehensive public health program.[5] Gottheil's sister, Eva Leon, who had also returned from a recent visit to Eretz Israel, reported on the immediate need for establishing maternity services in Jerusalem.[6]

Since the founding meeting of the organization took place during the Purim holiday, it was decided to call the new organization "Hadassah" — the Hebrew name for the heroine of the Purim story, Queen Esther. Henrietta Szold was elected president of the organization, together with a directorate of 19 women. The plan put forward by the organization was designed to encompass a daycare nursery, a lace-making workshop for girls, a maternity hospital, and a school for midwives and the operation of a regional program for nurses' training.

The Character of Hadassah as an Organization

Hadassah was established as a Zionist-philanthropic organization. Ben-Gurion commented at the time that "it is hard to know whether the suckling was more philanthropic or more Zionist."[7] A unique organization of American women for its time, Hadassah was structurally a new kind of Zionist framework — nonpartisan, void of a particular political line and above party politics.

Alon Gal, a scholar of American Jewry, claims that Hadassah is a distinctly American-Jewish organization — "made in America," so to speak. The organization arose and crystallized in the Progressive Era of American history (1890–1920) when feminism was one of the manifestations of progressivism, epitomized by women gaining the right to vote in 1920. Gal claims that combination of these two elements — progressivism and feminism, labeled in historical tracts as "social feminism" — constituted one of the underpinnings of Hadassah as an organization and has guided its activities throughout its existence. As a result, Hadassah developed as a social feminist–Zionist organization. Its members — like the progressives who operated in poor neighborhoods — aspired to work "on behalf of a healthy population that can properly cope on a personal and public level and towards a society that will make comely mothers and contented children a possibility."[8]

In June 1914, Hadassah organized a national convention in Rochester, New York. At this convention, the organization adopted a motto taken from Jeremiah — "Arucat Bat-Ami" (Healing of the Daughter of my People)[9] — and its symbol, a six-pointed Star of David emblazoned with the name of the organization and the biblical phrase. At the same gathering it was decided to join Hadassah's male counterpart, the Federation of American Zionists, a decision that was carried out only in 1918 when the latter changed its name to the Zionist Organization of America (ZOA). Henrietta Szold, who had taken upon herself to head the Organization's Education Department, believed that in the wake the Balfour Declaration, there was no point in a separate women's organization. She believed that at this juncture in time, it was befitting that American Zionists join together and speak "with one voice."[10]

But unity within the Zionist movement was short-lived. Ideological divisions broke out in 1921 during the ZOA's convention in Cleveland, Ohio. Dispute broke out between the American "pragmatic Zionists" camp lead by judge Louis Brandeis, and members of the European "political Zionist" camp headed by Dr. Chaim Weizmann, president of the World Zionist Organization (WZO). The "Brandeis group" claimed that the political mission of Zionism had been achieved with the publication of the Balfour Declaration — a public document issued in 1917 by British Foreign Secretary Lord Balfour that expressed British sympathy with

Jewish Zionist aspirations. The "Brandeis group" argued that the Zionist Organization should clarify its operations and concentrate on organizing Zionists worldwide and focusing on funding settlement activity and economic development in Eretz Israel. Weizmann, on the other hand, maintained that political Zionism was still in its infancy, and the World Zionist Organization must remain united behind active encouragement of Jewish immigration to Eretz Israel and mobilization of necessary capital for absorption of immigrants.

Hadassah found itself in the crossfire between the two camps: Brandeis' group on one side, Weizmann's supporters on the other. Most of the Hadassah delegates supported Brandeis' position, but the organization abstained from identifying with either camp.

At the Cleveland convention, Hadassah leadership learned that joining the Zionist Organization of America embroiled them in political frictions and limited their control over projects and funding that Hadassah was mobilizing. Henrietta Szold convinced her companions to cease the transfer of donations to the ZOA and to channel them directly towards the realization of Hadassah's special social welfare program in Eretz Israel.

Indeed, at the 1921 Hadassah convention in Pittsburgh, delegates voted in favor of autonomy and took over complete control of monies and programs. Passage of this resolution signaled the beginning of a process whereby Hadassah severed its organizational ties as part of the ZOA — a process that was completed in 1933 when Hadassah Women received total organizational freedom. Since then, Hadassah has been careful to preserve complete internal autonomy[11] and has continued to maintain its stature as a large, stable and highly organized independent body within American Zionism. Throughout the years, Hadassah has been marked by continual growth, in contrast with its male counterpart; the ZOA continued to suffer from ideological and organizational crises.[12]

Hadassah's "historical achievement" was in being "the first framework to succeed in genuinely interesting a large proportion of American Jewish women in involvement on behalf of Eretz Israel, presenting them with the option of social welfare improvements as a special area of endeavor. It is impossible to write the history of American Zionism — or Zionism in general — without citing the value of Hadassah as a core multifaceted agent in Zionist endeavors."[13]

The Outset of Hadassah Activity in Eretz Israel

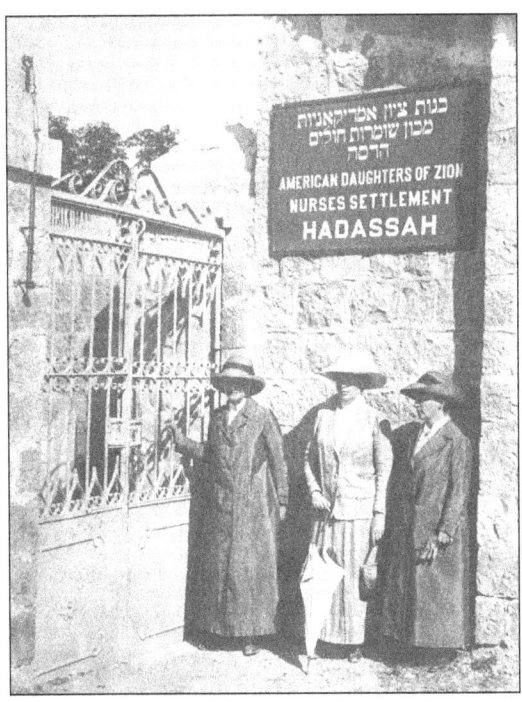

Rachel Landy (left) and Rose Kaplan (right), the first nurses sent by Hadassah to Eretz Israel, at the gate of the Nurses' Settlement in Mea Shearim (suburb) in Jerusalem. In the center: Eva Leon, one of the founders of Hadassah, Jerusalem 1913 (Courtesy of Hadassah Archives, NY).

Hadassah's activity began, in essence, on January 1, 1913. Members of the Hadassah directorate were called to a meeting, at which they were informed that the Jewish philanthropist Nathan Straus[14] expressed his consent to underwrite employment of a nurse to be chosen by Hadassah and sent to Jerusalem to establish a community nursing system. Nathan Straus was aware of this necessity; in 1912 he had visited Jerusalem, and had established a soup kitchen and health station. Straus urged Henrietta Szold to apply a regional scheme of nursing services for home visits to care for mothers and children, along the lines of those operating successfully in New York.[15] The Hadassah directorate approved Nathan Straus' plan and two nurses — Rose Kaplan and Rachel Landy — sailed for Eretz Israel.

On March 23, 1913, the two nurses arrived in Jerusalem — on the eve of the outbreak of World War I. The situation in Eretz Israel was horrendous and their training as nurses had not prepared them for the dire distress they encountered. Living conditions were harsh. The levels of sanitation and hygiene were extremely poor. Families lived in abject poverty, subject to hunger and malnutrition, disease and epidemics. The mortality rate among the elderly, the orphaned and the young was rampant. The outbreak of World War I in 1914 only added to the wretchedness of the Jewish community.

Cooperation that had existed between the Turkish government and the Jewish population in Eretz Israel at the outset of the war was short-lived. Following the arrival of Gamal pascha supreme commander of Turkish Forces, in Eretz Israel in November 1914, attitudes toward the Jewish population became harsh and hostile. The situation continued to deteriorate and terrorization of the population increased. Jews — suspected of being a hostile element — were subject to mistreatment, restrictive edicts and deportation.

American Jewry constituted the primary source of resources during this trying period, due to the neutralism of the United States during most of the war, a status that enabled them to send money, medications and food to the Jewish community in Eretz Israel.

The American Jewish Committee coordinated activities such as the collection of donations and their allocation for educational purposes in Eretz Israel. Massive assistance was provided to the population by Nathan Straus' health station that, in collaboration with Hadassah and the Eretz Israel Office (the Israeli branch office of the World Zionist Organization), organized the doctors in Jerusalem to establish the Medical Aid Committee (Va'ad HaEzrah Hameditzinit). This new committee provided free medical care in the homes of residents for patients left without treatment and medical assistance due to the shortage of hospital beds.

With the conquest of Eretz Israel by British forces in 1917, centuries of Ottoman rule came to an end. Introduction of British administrative culture brought about significant improvement in health and sanitation. Health clinics were established and the operation of existing hospital facilities was renewed. New undertakings in preventive medicine — such as the eradication of malaria and infectious diseases and improvements in hygiene, food and water quality — were made a top priority. Moreover, medical services for the indigent were opened. With the establishment of civilian government, a Health Department was organized, headed by Colonel George Wickham Heron who had led British health services in Egypt in 1908–1915. Colonel Heron subsequently headed the British Mandate's Health Department over the next two decades.[16]

The 1917 Balfour Declaration brought about a change of status for the Jewish community in Eretz Israel — or as it was called by the Zionists, "the Yishuv" (the Community). In 1918, the Zionist Commission in Jewish Palestine (Va'ad Hatzirim) — a core Zionist body led by Dr. Chaim Weizmann that was designed to initiate Jewish settlement and development projects in Eretz Israel — was established. Together with the Eretz Israel Office of the World Zionist Organization, the Commission took steps toward the development of a Hebrew educational network. Indeed, during Dr. Weizmann's tenure, education enjoyed priority over other areas in Zionist funding.

At the close of World War I, the Yishuv was destitute. Part of the population had died from disease, epidemics and famine. Families were uprooted from their homes. Thousands of widows and orphans were left in dire conditions without the means to sustain themselves. In the face of such a horrendous situation, the World Zionist Organization was forced to turn to the Zionist Organization of America to request aid. The latter assigned Hadassah with the mission since Hadassah was already engaged in philanthropic work in Eretz Israel. Hadassah — with the assistance of the non-Zionist American Jewish Joint Distribution Committee, a rescue and relief organization established in 1914 by the Zionist activist Otto Warburg — organized a medical mission, the American Zionist Medical Unit (AZMU) that included doctors, nurses, midwives and other health officers. AZMU brought with it modern medical equipment including ambulances and other vehicles, and medication. Immediately upon arrival in Eretz Israel in August 1918, the mission began medical-rehabilitative activity among the general population, founded upon principals set forth by Hadassah — "never to discriminate between Jew and Arab." The work of AZMU constituted the first bona fide infrastructure for preventive medicine, public hygiene and health education in Eretz Israel.

No other project in the history of Hadassah has had the same massive effect on the evolving character of the organization as the American Zionist Medical Unit. In 1921, on the foundations of AZMU, the Hadassah Medical Organization was established. The Organization was a framework dedicated solely to building a public health apparatus in Eretz Israel. Its scope encompassed a war on infant mortality, rehabilitation of hospitals, assistance to new mothers, improvement of hygiene and sanitation in educational institutions and attention to health needs of students in the school system. Today, the Hadassah Medical Organization directs all medical work of Hadassah, allocating the lion's share of the organization's budget to these areas.

The study to which this volume is dedicated covers the period of the British Mandate — from the arrival of AZMU operating under Hadassah auspices, until the establishment of the State of Israel — at which time Hadassah's health facilities were transferred to the newly established Ministry of Health. During this thirty-year period, Hadassah established — from scratch — a public health system on behalf of the welfare of mothers and children, founded upon a heightened awareness that recognition of the health needs of the child is a cornerstone for a mentally and physically healthy population.

The Ministry of Health of the State of Israel, which in 1948 "inherited" the health system built by Hadassah, continued to develop the Israeli health system along the lines set forth by Hadassah. Today, the public health system provides health services in all educational institutions and Family Health Stations operate throughout the country — mandated by law under the country's Compulsory Health Insurance Law. In content and spirit, the prevailing health system constitutes an authentic sequel to health services as conceived, created and operated by Hadassah during the Mandate period.

This study is based primarily on archival material — a mass of documents, protocols and reports from the early years of Hadassah in Eretz

Israel — preserved in the Central Zionist Archives (CZA) and Hadassah archives in New York City. In addition, the Labor Archives at the Lavon Institute in Tel Aviv (LA) contain important historical material on the relationship between Hadassah and the Federation of Labor's Sick Fund, Kupat Holim Ha'Clalit (The General Sick Fund), henceforth referred to as Kupat Holim.[17] Alongside archival material, the personal diaries and correspondence of figures of the period and media coverage at the time — as well as contemporary research by others — provided important sources of information as well.

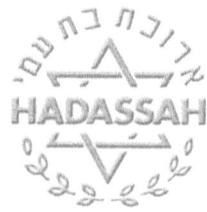

Chapter II

The American Zionist Medical Unit

World War I left the Yishuv in Eretz Israel isolated from sources
of financial support from abroad. This fact led to the deterioration of
the economic state of the community and the health of its inhabitants.
Medical attention was particularly distressed. Turkish military authorities
commandeered most hospitals and drug supplies, and many physicians
were drafted into the army. In mid-1916, a typhus epidemic broke out,
spreading rapidly, particularly in population centers. In Jerusalem, Jaffa
and Safed the epidemic caused the death of thousands, coupled with
additional victims of famine, other diseases and simple lack of proper
medical treatment.[18]

In July 1916, the Zionist Executive Committee *(Va'ad Hapoel Hazioni)*
— temporarily quartered in Copenhagen for the duration of the war —
approached the Histadruth of American Zionists requesting organization
of immediate medical aid for the Yishuv in Eretz Israel. Execution of the
request was assigned to the Zionist Women's Federation — Hadassah —
a natural choice reflecting the organization's work in public health in
Eretz Israel, going back to 1913. Hadassah began to organize a medical
delegation to assist the Yishuv. However, due to the United States' entrance
into the war in 1917, activity came to a standstill. American citizens were
not allowed to enter Eretz Israel; consequently, plans were postponed. In
December 1917, a short time after the liberation of Jerusalem by the British,

Hadassah members initiated contact with the British military government in order to gain permission for the American Zionist Medical Unit to enter Eretz Israel. Approval was received only in March 1918, following the personal intervention of Judge Louis Brandeis, who was aware of the immense importance of extending immediate medical assistance to rehabilitate the Jewish community.

Mobilization of American Zionists to assist the Yishuv stemmed from a number of reasons:

> The Zionist Commission of the World Zionist Organization headed by Dr. Chaim Weizmann arrived in Eretz Israel in 1918. They found that the American Red Cross was already there. Under the auspices of the British Foreign Office, the Red Cross was engaged in extending medical aid. The Commission feared that the Red Cross intended to launch ongoing activity in the country and saw this activity as a possible guise for introducing foreign elements into Eretz Israel. Therefore, immediate Zionist-Jewish action was called for, to obstruct such a move by the Red Cross.[19]

> Judge Louis Brandeis, chairman of the Ad-Hoc Executive Committee for Zionist Affairs (Va'ad Hapoel Hazmani Leinyanim Zioni'im) during World War I, aspired to take over leadership of the World Zionist Federation, at the time in the hands of Dr. Weizmann. For this reason, Brandeis encouraged American Zionists to demonstrate strenuous political activity vis-à-vis issues pertaining to Eretz Israel. Brandeis, who had visited the country and had been affected by the arduous state of the Yishuv, employed his personal esteem on behalf of the mobilization of funding to obtain the medical assistance needed.

> Unlike Jewish communities in Europe, American Jewry was the only Jewish community that had not been directly affected by the war. Thus, only American Jewry was relatively financially well off and able to bear financing medical assistance to the Yishuv.

> Assigning Hadassah with execution of the mission was an obvious choice since Hadassah members were already involved in philanthropic activity in Israel —within the organization's own limitations as defined by Henrietta Szold, who had said: "No alms! We are going to Israel equipped

*with the social-philanthropic work experience of American Jewish women;
our aim is to bring the achievements of American medicine to Israel...If
we can bring order to this land of chaos, no one will be able to accuse us
of being a benevolent society."[20]*

*On June 11, 1918, the American Zionist Medical Unit (hereafter "the
Unit") set out for Eretz Israel under Hadassah auspices. The medical team
was composed of 44 physicians (specialists in dermatology, ophthalmology,
gynecology, orthopedics, pathology, and ENT), 20 nurses (the oldest a
mere 25 years old), pharmacists, medical assistants, personnel in medical
administration, accompanied by modern medical equipment valued at
more than $25,000[21] — half of which was underwritten by the American
Joint Distribution Committee.[22] Additional physicians with suitable
medical training to complete the medical team were mobilized in Europe,
or in Eretz Israel proper. All members of the Unit were volunteers. On one
hand, many had never been beyond the borders of the United States and
lacked any experience in rendering medical assistance under emergency
conditions such as those in Israel. On the other hand, the readiness of all
to partake in the mission was tremendous. Dr. Isaac Max Rubinow was
appointed medical director and chief administrator, in charge of operation
of the Unit in Eretz Israel. Dr. Rubinow, however, announced just prior to
the departure of the Unit that for personal reasons he would not be able
to accompany the Unit. Dr. Rubinow promised to join them without delay,
and indeed arrived in Israel — in March 1919.[23]*

Dr. Isaac Max Rubinow

Dr. Isaac Max Rubinow (1875–1936) was born in Russia and
immigrated to the United States in 1893. He received his medical training
at New York University and for five years worked as a neighborhood doctor
among poor immigrant populations on the Lower East Side. Afterwards,
he studied sociology and statistics. Influenced by his studies and his
experiences among the poor, Dr. Rubinow became active in promoting
social legislation, particularly in the field of health legislation. He argued

that compulsory health insurance legislation was the only solution to the distress of the lower classes in health matters. Impressed by European social legislation that developed at the end of the nineteenth century — particularly health insurance laws in Germany and England — Dr. Rubinow lobbied on behalf of similar legislation in the United States within the framework of the American Association for Labor Legislation (AALL).[24] The Association, established at the onset of World War I, included physicians, public servants and political leaders who espoused social reform. A good number of them, including Dr. Rubinow, were confessed socialists.[25]

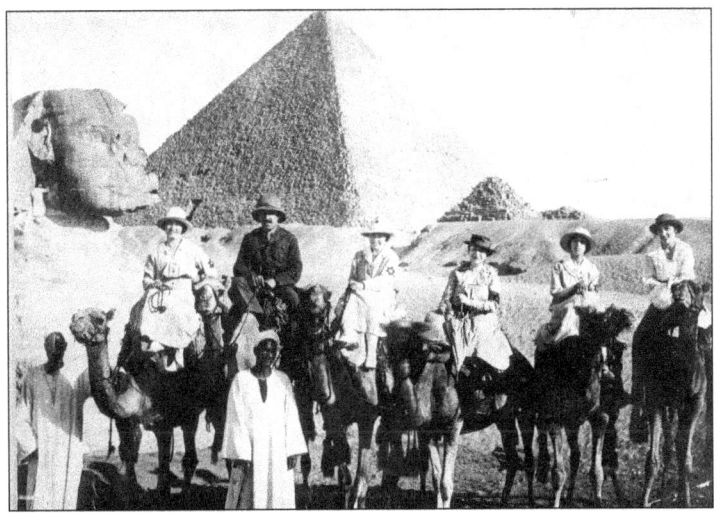

Nurses from the Medical Unit, Hadassah, near the Pyramids, in their way to Eretz Israel, July 1918 (Courtesy of Hadassah Archives, NY).

The appointment of Dr. Rubinow as director of the Unit came in the wake of failure of the AALL to bring about passage of broad-based social legislation in the United States, particularly a compulsory health insurance law. Dr. Rubinow had been one of the leaders of this struggle. Prior to his Hadassah appointment, Dr. Rubinow had not been close to Jewish matters, nor was he at all active in Zionist affairs during eight years of activism on behalf of the AALL. The United States' entrance into World

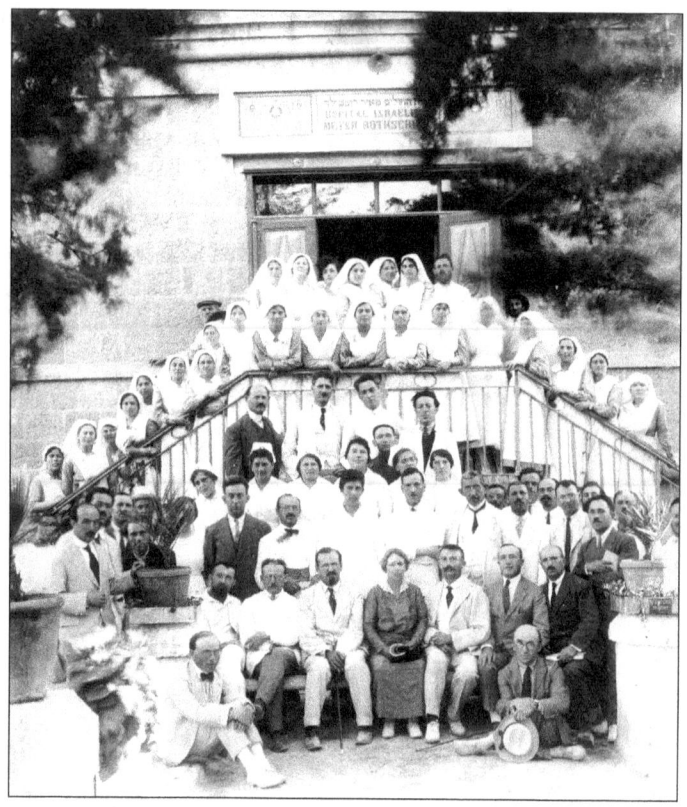

*American Zionist Medical Unit, Hadassah, 1919, Jerusalem
(Donchin-Hadassah Collection).*

War I in 1917 sparked a wave of anti-German activity that encompassed
even those who had been active in favor of social legislation along the
lines of German compulsory health legislation. As a result, the operations
of the AALL came to a standstill. Dr. Rubinow was even accused of being
a traitor and German sympathizer, was banished from all key posts and
found himself unemployed. The American Medical Association, riddled
with anti-Semitism, blocked any possibility for integration of Jewish
doctors within university institutions. Even the federal government,
which had employed Dr. Rubinow before the war, now refrained from
employing him. One may assume that the failure of the struggle to pass

a compulsory health insurance law in the United States, coupled with the damage to Dr. Rubinow's professional career as a result of anti-German sentiment, prompted Dr. Rubinow to agree when queried by Henrietta Szold if he would be willing to take upon himself administration of the American Zionist Medical Unit being organized and carried out under Hadassah auspices. Acceptance of the post constituted a positive solution to Dr. Rubinow's economic quandary and allowed him to continue to practice medicine. Moreover, the post gave Dr. Rubinow an opportunity to try and apply some of his ideas about how health services should be structured and organized in the United States — in Eretz Israel.[26]

Range of Activity of the American Zionist Medical Unit

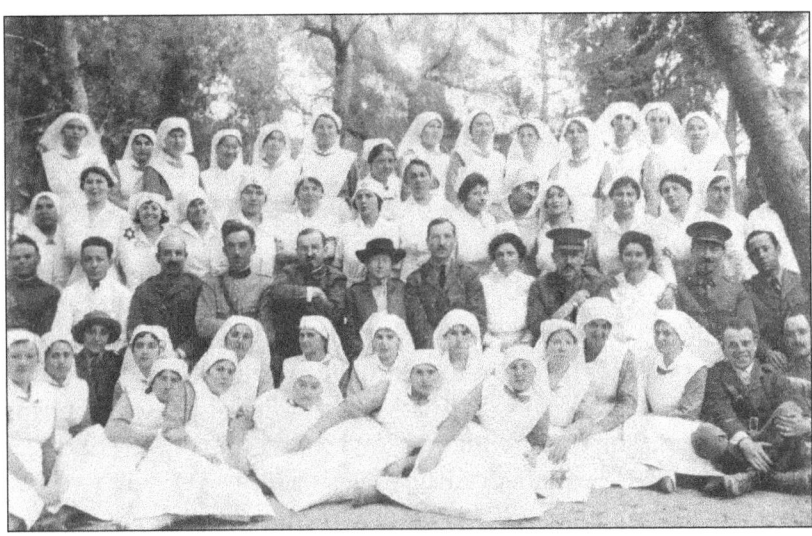

American Zionist Medical Unit, Jerusalem 1920s (Donchin-Hadassah Collection).

Upon their arrival in Eretz Israel in August 1918, the Unit was initially totally occupied with urgent medical issues; only toward the end of the year, in November 1918, was the Unit able to turn its attention to opening hospitals in urban centers. The Unit renewed operation of the main hospital in Jerusalem — the Rothschild Hospital — and transformed the facility into the Unit's headquarters in Eretz Israel. Concurrently, the Unit reopened the community hospital in Jaffa — Sha'ar Zion Hospital — that had been closed at the end of the war due to a financial crisis stemming from lack of funding.[27] New hospitals were founded in Tiberias and Haifa, and a tuberculoses sanitarium was opened in Safed. Adjacent to each hospital, a clinic and laboratory was established. Unit policy stipulated that payment for hospitalization would be based on the ability of each individual patient to pay; indigent patients were fully exempt. Adoption of such a policy was based on the principals that traditionally guided Jewish mutual aid societies — a fundamental and integral part of Jewish community life and social culture regarding care of poor patients.[28]

In order to overcome the shortage of professionally trained heath workers, the Unit opened a nursing school adjacent to the Rothschild-Hadassah Hospital in Jerusalem, formulating a unique curriculum for nurses' training based on modern nursing principles, in accordance with teaching curriculums employed at the time in the United States. In addition, instruction was given to graduate nurses to adapt their professional outlook to the nature of work and the special needs of the local population.

The Unit's Nurses' School was the first of its kind in Eretz Israel. The administrative and teaching staff was placed in the hands of certified nurses serving in the Unit. The student body was composed partially of newly arrived Zionist-oriented immigrants, partially of native-born young women — some of who had previously worked as practical nurses in hospitals and local clinics. The first graduating class was witness to the outbreak of Arab riots of 1921. A number of nurses were sent to Tel Aviv to organize an emergency hospital for victims of the violence.[29] Other graduates were sent to hospitals, clinics, agricultural settlements and encampments of road-builders and swamp-drainage projects — laying the foundations for professional and orderly nursing services throughout the Yishuv. [30]

Training of professional health workers became a precondition for any attempt to expand the Unit's activities — particularly expansion into rural areas suffering from malaria and in need of improved sanitation and preventive medicine. The Unit received authorization to operate from British mandatory authorities; throughout all its years of service, the British refrained from intruding in the affairs of the Unit, giving it total independence in running its operations. Concurrently, the Unit also received administrative support from the World Zionist Organization — support that allowed the Unit to demand and receive the compliance of the Yishuv regarding working principles set forth by the Unit itself.

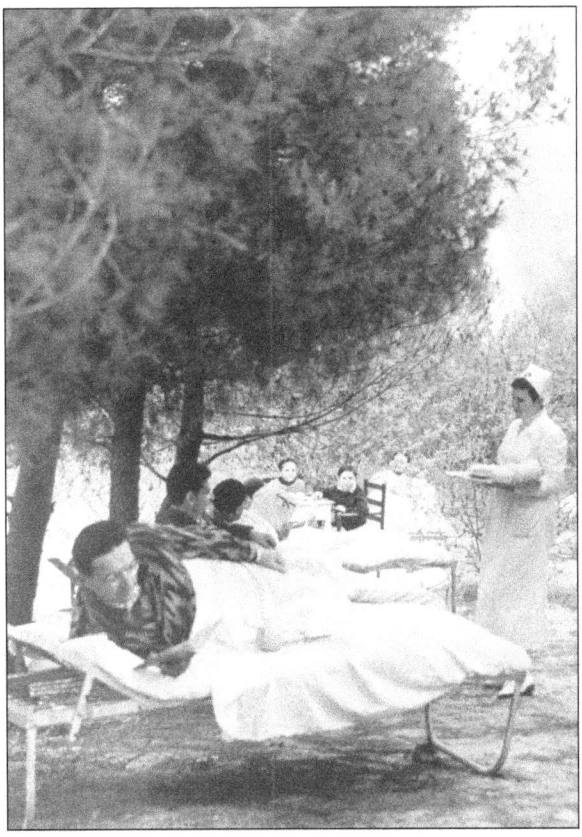

Hadassah senatorium for TB patients in the Galilee region (Donchin-Hadassah Collection).

The arrival of the Unit and its early operations was positively received by the Yishuv and its institutions. The Jewish community expected that within a short time, improvement in harsh health realities would be felt. This atmosphere was described in detail by educator Zeev Carmi in his autobiography *An Educator and His Way*:

> *Our guests — a group of physicians in British army uniforms, who showed up within days of the conquest of the city [Tiberias], generated tremendous rejoicing and a sense of national pride. They presented themselves as delegates of an American Jewish organization called Hadassah that was accompanying the conquest in order to survey the health situation in the Yishuv and to set up medical assistance. The city was filled with refugees from the deportation[31] and sanitary conditions and hygiene inferior by any standard. One of the doctors among the guests, Dr. Norman, who speaks Hebrew, remained and began organizing modern medical assistance like in America.[32]*

Kupat Holim, together with the Hebrew Medical Association, immediately made contacts with the Unit to update them on the prevailing health situation and to create a setup for collaboration between all parties in the health field.[33] Local Israeli doctors gave Unit physicians detailed reports on mortality in urban centers and villages and conducted orientation tours of existing medical facilities. The local medical community hoped that the arrival of the Unit would enhance their own shaky economic straits by providing additional opportunities for employment for physicians.

Policy, Structure and Organization of the Unit's Operations

In March 1919, Dr. Rubinow arrived in Eretz Israel and took over administration of the Unit. Doron Netherland wrote:

> *The medical delegation led by Rubinow wrote on its banner the total socialization of medical services. Therefore, the Unit began establishing a centralist medical service based on a national network of hospitals and clinics — all subordinate to the central administration of the organization.[34]*

In order to make the Unit's work more efficient, the country was divided into five regions. Directors of regional hospitals were appointed as heads of each region in order to coordinate work between the clinics and the hospital. As compensation, the hospital directors received a bonus to their salaries for this administrative role. All the regions were subordinate to the direct supervision of the Unit's administration and the Medical Center in Jerusalem.

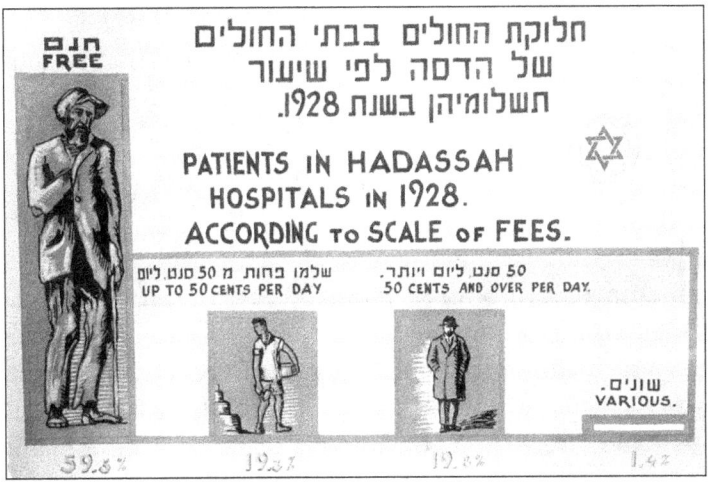

Patients in Hadassah Hospitals in 1928 according
to Scale of Fees (Donchin-Hadassah Collection).

Dr. Rubinow argued that the core precondition for full socialization of medical services was a fundamental change in the structure of the physicians' work — in other words, the replacement of private practice with salaried physicians practicing within the framework of public health organizations.[35]

Consequently, Dr. Rubinow passed a landmark regulation that was destined to put its stamp on the development of the character of the Unit's work and that of the Hadassah Medical Federation: "The regulation stipulates in regard to doctors — that they give all their time to their posts."[36] According to this regulation, Unit physicians were forbidden from engaging in private practice, under the rationale that they must dedicate all their time to their posts, and receive adequate salaries for a livelihood. Permission to engage in private practice would lead to negligence in fulfilling their roles in hospitals and polyclinics.[37] Moreover, each physician was required to agree to be posted wherever the Unit sent him. Failure to accept a particular post without adequate reason was grounds for immediate dismissal. In Dr. Rubinow's view, this regulation was designed to introduce a dimension of egalitarianism into the health system, and prevent situations whereby those of means would be favored in receipt of medical services. In order to further enhance equality in receipt of treatment, Dr. Rubinow further stipulated that patients would not be able to choose their physician. The aim was to create a service system wherein all doctors would serve all patients, without discrimination between rich and poor. In this manner, health services would be equal to all.[38] In setting up such a system of operation, Dr. Rubinow designed to apply in practice the idea of public medicine in its purest form.

Centralism of control and supervision were the primary characteristics of the Unit's preventive medicine plan. In order to prevent the spread of disease by new immigrants and gain a comprehensive picture of their health status, the Unit opened temporary guesthouses in the Jaffa Port where newcomers were sent upon arrival. During their sojourn, immigrants were required to undergo medical checkups by Unit doctors. They were examined, administered immunization shots where required, and given instruction on matters of hygiene, nutrition and sanitation. To prevent evasion of checkups, the Unit demanded that the Immigration Bureau — a local body responsible for processing the absorption of new immigrants — withhold food and lodging from those without documentation proving that they had undergone a medical checkup as required.[39] In this manner, Dr. Rubinow and his colleagues hoped that they would be able to supervise the health of the Yishuv, protect inhabitants from contagious diseases and bring about improvement in the general health of the community.

Dr. Rubinow held that the Unit should not engage solely in medical supervision, but should also play a part in the provision of welfare services for the Yishuv. According to his outlook, health work cannot operate if isolated from social welfare issues. To meet this challenge one needed to establish a central public organization to supervise and direct these services. In keeping with this conceptual approach, in 1919 the Unit established a School Hygiene Department under the direction of Dr. Mordechai Berachiahu to monitor and supervise the health of kindergarten and school children in the Yishuv.[40]

The School Hygiene Department first operated in Jerusalem. In 1920, its scope of operations was expanded to encompass four other major cities. Hygienic supervision also included schools in nearby settlements and agricultural villages in the vicinity. Supervision was provided to the schools gratis and funded by the Unit itself. The program focused on teaching hygiene, supervision of sanitation hygiene within the school and preventive treatment of skin and eye diseases — mainly ringworm and trachoma. The latter disease, a source of blindness if left untreated, was prevalent among children in Eretz Israel at the time. Concurrent to supervision of children in the schools, the Unit also opened Mother & Child Health Centers to provide pregnant women and new mothers with supervision and instruction in the raising of their infants. In this manner, the Unit hoped to educate mothers according to American standards of child rearing, based on knowledge of proper nutrition, attention to the infants weight and physical exercise — thus enhancing the health of children and reducing child mortality.

Centralist Administration and American Standards

The centralist structure of the Unit's operation and Dr. Rubinow's emphatic insistence on maintenance of high professional norms customary in the United States, soon led to clashes between the indigenous medical community and the Unit's physicians. Dr. Hillel Yaffe — director of the hospital in Zichron Yaakov and a leading figure in the physicians' professional organization, the Hebrew Medical Federation in Eretz Israel — noted that the Unit's physicians put little stock in the broad practical experience gained by members of the local medical community; declined to involve the Yishuv's doctors in their operations; related to local physicians with arrogance; and belittled all that had been done and achieved in health matters prior to their arrival.[41] On the other hand, members of the Unit argued that their seemingly cold attitude and aloofness toward local doctors stemmed from their desire to maintain —

at all costs — the high levels of expertise and medical standards they had brought with them from America.

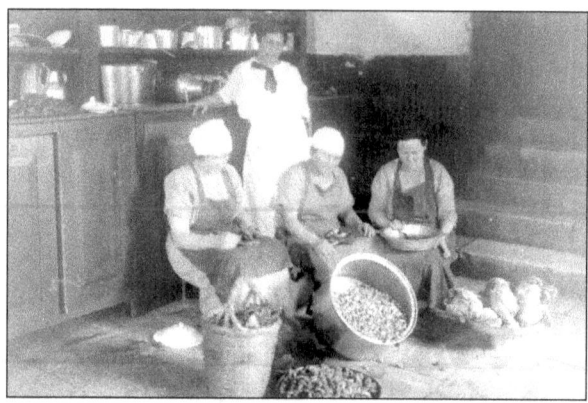

Hadassah nurse supervised the food preparation in Hadassah hospital in Jerusalem. Cleanliness and sanitation were major issues of Hadassah nurses work (Donchin-Hadassah Collection).

NUMBER OF PATIENTS מספר החולים
ADMITTED TO שנתקבלו 3481 1919
HADASSAH לבתי החולים 4673 1920
HOSPITALS. של הדסה. 5192 1921
6936 1922
7880 1923
8330 1924
9708 1925
10041 1926
10334 1927
10369 1928

Number of parents admitted to Hadassah hospitals in Jerusalem, Tel Aviv, and Haifa (Donchin-Hadassah Collection).

Dr. Rubinow himself admitted that the arrival of the Unit had placed local doctors in a difficult position: "I must admit just how grave the situation of doctors outside the Unit is. They found themselves pushed onto the sidelines professionally by those who have come from America. Not only their professional stature but also their income has suffered; some can barely eke out a living."[42] Dr. Hillel Yaffe bore witness to the same: "A number of long-standing physicians in the Yishuv whose education and experience is several times the mediocre education of American doctors, remain without work and with nothing to do because all the inhabitants go to Hadassah."[43]

In addition to clashes between Unit physicians and local physicians, a labor dispute also developed between Unit doctors and Unit management. The crux of the dispute focused on work arrangements and pay schedules formulated by Dr. Rubinow for Unit physicians, including internal dissension over whether senior physicians should be allowed to engage in private practice in addition to the practice of public medicine. Furthermore, complaints of discrimination among patients by Unit physicians were raised in the local Hebrew press.[44] In the wake of such criticism, Dr. Rubinow sent a report to Hadassah management in the United States explaining that "complaints about lack of care were raised by many patients. While many of the cases were found to be baseless, public opinion had to be coped with. Patients who did not pay for private service often felt that patients who could afford to pay for private service received better service."[45] Attempts by Dr. Rubinow to answer accusations through the press and explain Unit policy only exacerbated the tense relations.

Volatile relationships among Unit doctors themselves, among Unit doctors and their patients, and Unit doctors and the Yishuv's veteran physicians were present during the entire period in which Dr. Rubinow directed the Unit's affairs — even after 1921 when the Unit underwent organizational change with the inauguration of the Hadassah Medical Federation, under Rubinow's leadership.

Clashes over Management and Financing in Health Services within the Yishuv

In mid-1919, differences of opinion arose between the World Zionist Organization and the Unit. The Zionist Commission of the World Zionist Organization, headed by Menachem Ussishkin — a body comprised of prominent Jews, dispatched on the initiative of the British government in 1918 to survey the situation in Eretz Israel and make plans for the future — found itself embroiled in the conflict. Ussishkin viewed himself as a sort of WZO "trustee" vis-à-vis the work of the Unit in Eretz Israel, based on administrative authority granted him by the Zionist Federation and British authorities. Dr. Rubinow and members of the Unit argued that it was proper that the Unit's work be autonomous — administered directly and only by the Zionist Women's Federation, Hadassah. The Unit's demand for autonomy, while supported by the American Zionist Federation, was categorically rejected by members of the labor movement in Eretz Israel. Their position was clearly expressed in the *Hapoel Hatzair* newspaper:

The sharp language employed in the *Hapoel Hatzair* editorial against the Unit reflects intense animosities harbored by workers toward the Unit. The Unit was perceived as a body that pursued solely its own self-interests while ignoring the general Zionist interest, and was considered an arrogant body that viewed the Yishuv in Eretz Israel as an inferior element unaware of its own genuine needs that must be taught proper manners. Hapoel Hatzair even suggested boycotting Dr. Rubinow and the Unit in response to its arrogant attitude and desires to operate independent of and in isolation from the Yishuv's own institutions.

To understand the attitude of the Unit toward calls for assistance from the workers, one should stress the fundamental fact that the workers' organizations in 1919–20 numbered only a few thousand members, including those who were tied to Kupat Holim — at most 3,000 persons.[46] In comparison with the overall Yishuv — some 57,000 souls at the end of 1918 — the group was not considered to be particularly important, and certainly not of the magnitude that would justify channeling special medical assistance to them, beyond their proportional weight in the general population. Members of the Unit treated the workers relative to the size of the population they belonged to. The fact that leaders of the Yishuv during this period — figures such as David Ben-Gurion, Yitzhak Ben-Zvi and Berl Katznelson — were members of workers' groups and their political and social influence, while very significant, did not sway Unit policy regarding allocation of resources. The state of the urban Yishuv was no better off from a health standpoint than the plight of the workers in the encampments and agricultural settlements. In fact, the health situation in Jerusalem was even worse. Therefore, Dr. Rubinow's calculations — to ignore requests from the workers to a certain extent, and channel most of the Unit's capabilities to the urban population — were justified, and were not, as the workers believed, a case of purposeful detriment or callous disregard for the workers' needs. Despite their small numbers, the workers placed great value on themselves as the primary Zionist force — and in some cases the only force — seriously engaged in building Eretz Israel.[47] However, an organization such as the Unit that was detached from the local milieu and unaware of underlying political and social dynamics at play, could not relate to workers' organizations according to their achievements or their political potential. The Unit dealt with them by employing objective criteria: the number of members and the urgency of medical treatment. By these standards, the workers received no more and no less than what they were entitled.

Researchers of the period have suggested other undercurrents at work — personal as well as political.

Donald Miller in his work on Hadassah[48] wrote that power struggles and clashes over finances were an integral part of the general struggle over control of health services in Eretz Israel. This conflict was first concentrated in confrontations between the Unit and the Zionist Commission sent by the World Zionist Organization to survey conditions in Eretz Israel. Later, the conflict centered on strife between the Unit and the Health Committee established by the Yishuv at the beginning of the 1920s.[49] According to research conducted by Doron Niederland, it is possible to explain the conflicts as the direct result of the administrative-bureaucratic centralism upon which the workings of the Unit in the country was founded — centralism that was opposed by many elements in the Yishuv.[50] However, Daniel Fox, a scholar who researched the history of social medicine in the United States and examined the work of Dr. Rubinow in the United States, claims that many conflicts with Dr. Rubinow stemmed from the physician's rigid personality. Fox believes that Dr. Rubinow had difficulty forging normal working relationships based on cooperation and mutual trust. Demanding that everything be done his way, Dr. Rubinow carried out his business on a purely centralist and power-oriented basis. As a result, his management style and policies led to conflict with all those he encountered.[51]

A General Federation of Labor summary report published in 1921 describes the interrelationship between the workers and the Unit thus:

> *Until 1922, relationships between Hadassah [i.e., a referral to the Unit] and Kupat Holim were not orderly or enduring. There was no mutual agreement setting forth principles for a collaborative work framework. The consequences of this situation were immediately evident. Lack of a joint work program in locations and among groups where the two institutions opened operations, led to collision. One of the known sources [of conflict] was the fact that Hadassah as a strong medical federation with a large and dependable budget did not think it necessary to take the workers' mutual aide institution into consideration — an institution that had not yet consolidated and developed sufficiently. On one hand, these relationships resulted in expenditure of energy and resources needlessly, while on the other hand, groups of workers were forced to bear the burden of double expenses...If the budget that up until now was received and disbursed by Hadassah, would be delivered directly to us, this would have a great [positive] effect on the authority of the Sick Fund, on growth in membership and strengthen the Fund financially and economically. This would bring the institution closer to its goal — organization of rational and proper medical assistance based on mutual assistance, fully adapted to the requirements of the Yishuv and Jewish immigration.[52]*

The impression one gets from this report is that the Labor Federation accused the Unit of impairing the work of the Kupat Holim as a result of excessive strictness in money matters among Dr. Rubinow and his colleagues in the Unit, and due to Dr. Rubinow's aspirations to single-handedly set priorities for expenditures. The workers wanted to receive the Unit's financial assistance without preconditions — a demand the Unit did not accept.

The differing positions of the Unit and the Labor Federation over finances were the basis for harsh disputes throughout the 1920s.

From a Temporary Emergency Unit to Hadassah Medical Organization

In 1920, British military rule in the country was abolished and civilian Mandatory rule established. The change in government called for a change in the deployment and organization of the Unit. Between 1918 and 1920 the Unit operated as a temporary emergency framework whose goal was to dispense immediate medical assistance for urgent problems. With the onset of British civilian rule, the Unit was requested to assist in setting up a health system that would provide ongoing and permanent treatment for the Jewish community in the country. This mission, who was not suitable for a temporary organization, added one more reason in favor of the Unit personnel's demand that the Unit be transformed into a permanent and autonomous institution in its own right. After a year of deliberations, in September 1921, the 12th Zionist Congress held in Carlsbad decided to transform the Unit from a temporary organization into an independent health organization under the name Hadassah Medical Federation. It was stipulated in the decision that the Federation would operate autonomously, directly subordinate to the Zionist Women's Federation — Hadassah.[53]

Concurrently the Congress moved to establish a Yishuv Health Committee that would take upon itself organization, administration and coordination of all health operations within the Yishuv. In addition, the Zionist Congress demanded that the Unit formally adjust its ties with the workers' organizations within a contractual framework, in order to forestall further conflict. In mid-1922, the first work contract was signed between the Unit and Kupat Holim. According to the terms of the contract, the Unit — now known as the Hadassah Medical Federation — took upon itself to finance from the assistance budget of the Zionist Congress to Kupat Holim half the expenditures of Kupat Holim on medications and medical equipment. Secondly, the Hadassah Medical Federation agreed to provide hospitalization services to workers at a reduced rate. Hadassah even committed itself not to intervene in medical practices of Kupat Holim.[54]

The agreement that formalized the relationship between the Unit (i.e., Hadassah) and Kupat Holim, in essence, permanently institutionalized the principle of socialized health services in the country. Kupat Holim itself adopted Dr. Rubinow's fundamental perceptions regarding hygiene, instruction in proper nutrition, centralized supervision of the health of immigrants arriving in the country and the continued operation of Mother & Child Health Centers. Kupat Holim even opened health centers of its own in agricultural settlements, modeled after the Unit's Mother & Child Health Centers. Moreover, the Kupat Holim's doctors were required to work according to arrangements customary in Hadassah — in other words, medical practice based on salary only, prohibition of private practice and institution of a collective work contact.[55]

Toward the End of the Rubinow Era

Termination of the Unit's role as a temporary medical assistance organization on behalf of the Yishuv. and the organization of a permanent framework, the Hadassah Medical Federation, brought a turnabout in the work of Dr. Rubinow. Three intensive years of work accompanied by continuous budgetary constraints, disputes over private practice and quarrels with the workers that were marked by personal attacks in the local press, prompted Dr. Rubinow to leave the country and return to the United States. Henrietta Szold's repeated requests that he take upon himself management of the new organization were rejected. Dr. Rubinow was hurt and adamant to leave even before a replacement could be appointed. In a farewell speech before members of Hadassah prior to leaving the country, Dr. Rubinow expressed this in his address:

> *Those who know how to act under all circumstances are usually considered charming and cultured. But those who are always committing embarrassing mistakes who do and say the wrong things at the wrong times betray themselves as uncultured. I might as well confess that according to this commandment I have all too often betrayed myself as uncultured...I might have even made friends by learning Hebrew rather than working fourteen hours a day. So I failed in this. I was not popular with the staff because I put the needs of the people above those of the staff... and then having quarreled with the staff I proceeded to quarrel*

with all the powers in the Zionist movement... And having preserved the independence of the AZMU I proceeded to fight with the American organization and made many enemies there, because I insisted that our physicians must have no private practice...that did not stop the outside medical men from attacking me as of old. So I have not made many friends, did not get much gratitude...But I hope you will believe me if I say that my thoughts will always be with Palestine.[56]

Officially, Dr. Rubinow stepped down from his post in 1922 and returned to the United States, but Henrietta Szold's persistence paid off and he eventually agreed to return to Eretz Israel for an additional period to manage the Hadassah Medical Federation until a permanent director could be found. In 1923, Dr. Rubinow left for good and returned to the United States. Initially, he tried to reintegrate into the American medical establishment, but failed. In subsequent years, he worked as director of the American Zionist Federation, later receiving an appointment from Bnai Brith, where Dr. Rubinow worked until his death in 1936.

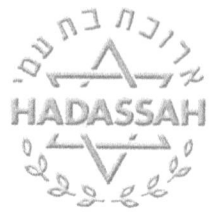

Chapter III

The School Hygiene Department

A. The Development of the School Hygiene Department

The First School Medical Services

Health and hygiene services for school children and supervision of sanitation in educational institutions began to develop in European countries and America in the nineteenth century. In France, Germany, Belgium, Sweden, England and the United States regular medical supervision of pupils began in the mid-nineteenth century. The primary goal was to prevent the spread of communicable diseases.[57]

In Israel, this process began only after World War I with the arrival of the Unit. In 1919 the Unit initiated establishment of a School Hygiene Department under its auspices. Up until that time, all schools in Israel lacked any hygiene supervision; the only exception was the Herzliya Gymnasium in Tel Aviv. From the time of its founding in 1908, the Herzliya Gymnasium employed a part-time physician on a permanent basis.[58] While the school doctor devoted most of his time to his private practice, the high school nonetheless enjoyed relatively good medical supervision. The school doctor was assigned responsibility not only for curative care of ill students but also ongoing hygiene that included a yearly checkup for each student; maintenance of health records on a personal health chart; weighing and measuring the height of students biannually; and suitable seating arrangements in the classroom based on individual eye examinations. Children suffering from trachoma — common ophthalmologic diseases among inhabitants of Eretz Israel at the time — were not accepted by the gymnasium at all; students who contracted the disease were suspended by the Herzliya Gymnasium until they were well. In other schools in Jerusalem and Tel Aviv, only preventive ophthalmologic care to treat trachoma among the student body was conducted.

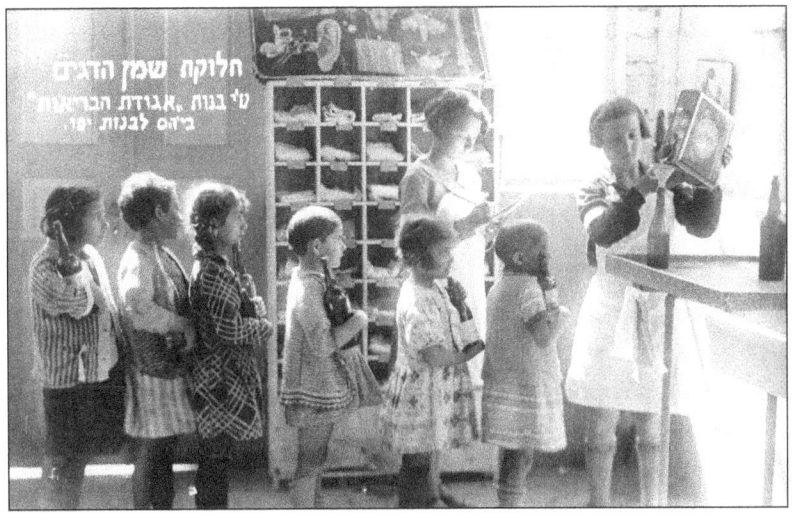

Delivering of fish oil for school children as part of Hadassah nutrition program to improve children health (Donchin-Hadassah Collection).

Curative treatment of trachoma was first adopted by the Girls' School in Jaffa on the initiative of the school principal, Mordechai Ckerishvsky-Ezrachi.[59] Diagnosis of those girls infected with the disease was carried out on school premises by a doctor, and a paramedic who administered daily treatment to students. In time, medical care became a regular, integral part of the general operation of the school, and pupils learned to take precautionary measures to protect the health of their eyes.

In 1909, Henrietta Szold visited Israel for the first time. Szold was appalled by the harsh situation prevailing in Jerusalem, Tiberias and Safed — particularly the terrible state of hygiene. In her estimation, poor hygiene constituted the primary factor affecting the health of both Jewish and Arab communities.[60] When Szold toured Jerusalem, the poverty and poor state of health of the inhabitants shocked her. Jerusalem in those days was a very squalid city; sewage ran in the streets and typhus and cholera epidemics spread readily. Most children were infected with skin and eye diseases, particularly ringworm and trachoma.

Isaiah Press, one of the first teachers in Jerusalem, vividly described the deplorable state of affairs in his book *A Hundred Years in Jerusalem:*

> *...Neglect in the city was widespread, and negligence permeated the life of the inhabitants. Sunrays almost didn't penetrate the narrow arched streets. Mildew grew on the streets and the walls of the houses. Sewage flowed in the courtyards of the houses and piles of garbage and carcasses at the sides of the streets raised a stench, harboring malaria germs that took their toll among the residents.*[61]

The unsound state of sanitation in the city and shortage of food and water, medical specialists and effective medications led to diseases that spread from house to house, courtyard to courtyard, becoming epidemics that swept away many victims. Mortality was particularly widespread among young children.

In her visit to Jaffa, Szold was particularly impressed by the work curing ophthalmologic diseases carried out in the Girls' School and decided to expand this endeavor. At her suggestion, Hadassah initiated treatment for ophthalmologic diseases in Jerusalem schools as well. This project was inaugurated in March 1913 by two nurses, Rose Kaplan and Rachel Landy, who were sent to Eretz Israel under the auspices of Hadassah and financed by the Jewish philanthropist Nathan Straus. The pair devoted most of their time to care of infants and treatment of trachoma. The two nurses coordinated their trachoma program with the renowned Jerusalem ophthalmologist, Dr. Avraham Ticho.[62]

The curative program continued throughout World War I, despite difficult wartime conditions. Work was organized and directed by an ophthalmologist, aided by a team of assistants who were specially trained for this task. Other than daily treatment of those pupils infected with trachoma, the physician also carried out periodic general checkups of the entire student body once every three months. In those days, other than ophthalmologic treatment, no other medical procedures were carried out in schools

Introduction of modern hygiene within the secular school network established by Zionist settlers, where the language of instruction was Hebrew, began only with the arrival of the Unit. The issue of student health and the need for supervisory policy regarding the health of the student body and hygienic-sanitary conditions within the confines of educational institutions were among the first missions that the Unit took upon itself to address. In fact, medical supervision of pupils constituted one of the most outstanding branches of Hadassah's constructive endeavors in Eretz Israel.

The choice of priorities was based on an acute awareness that care for the health of children was fundamental for a healthy population and the foundation for all progressive medicine. The severe health situation underscored the need to create a comprehensive and coherent method of effectively battling neglect and distress. It was clear that without education of children and parents, all attempts to improve their condition were doomed to fail. Therefore, among the first missions for which the Unit took responsibility was medical care in schools and kindergartens associated with the Education Committee[63] and the establishment of a School Hygiene Department. These were the first missions among many tackled by Hadassah in the field of preventive medicine, all of which reflected the aspirations of the organization to rise a new generation healthy in body and spirit.

Dr. Mordechai Berachiahu, the school physician at the Herzliya Gymnasium in Tel Aviv, was appointed head of the newly established School Hygiene Department. He served in that capacity between 1912 and 1919. During its first year, the Department operated solely in Jerusalem. Only in 1920 were activities expanded to schools in Tel Aviv and Haifa, rapidly covering all educational institutions throughout the country.

Status of the School Hygiene Department within the System of Governmental Bodies and Links between Them

The School Hygiene Department dedicated itself to inaugurating health services, hygiene and sanitation in educational institutions operating under the auspices of the National Committee (*Va'ad Haleumi*), the governing body of the Yishuv. The Unit's School Hygiene Department operated side by side with other health bodies: the Health Department of the Mandatory government, the Health Committee of the National Committee and the Kupat Holim of the Federation of Labor. Many disagreements arose between the School Hygiene Department and these other bodies — disagreements characterized by struggles for power and over allocation of authority that emanated from aspirations to control financial and human resources — rivalry that at times spilled over into violent verbal confrontations.

The monetary crises that struck the civilian Mandatory government in its first years and Hadassah in the 1930s changed budgetary priorities and shaped the state of public medicine in general, and the School Hygiene Department in particular.[64] Throughout its existence the Department struggled to receive funding, job slots for nurses and doctors, and improvements in salaries. Budget cuts forced upon the Department affected its ability to function and develop. More than once, this sparked conflict between the Department's director Dr. Berachiahu and his superiors. In addition to clashes over health matters and precedents, there were also clashes with the powers-that-be in the field of education.

The School Hygiene Department focused its operation on educational institutions operating under the auspices of the National Committee. Thus, along with bodies that engaged in public health, the School Hygiene Department was forced to cope with bodies that were in charge of education of the young generation, as the Education Committee and the Education Department, supervisors, principals, teachers and kindergarten teachers generally sought to be those deciding health matters although they were not professionally trained to do so.

The Hygiene Department vis-à-vis the Mandatory Health Department

With institution of civilian Mandatory government, relations marred by hostility and distrust developed between the Yishuv and the British Mandate's Government Health Department, headed by Colonel Heron.

The National Committee demanded that Mandatory authorities recognize the right of the Yishuv to establish an independent medical system, as a public system, and called for government participation in maintaining the system. Colonel Heron rejected this demand and cited that the government provided health services to all citizens without discrimination, stressing the wasteful character of Jewish health services, particularly Hadassah's, in comparison with frugal conditions and economy prevailing in his own government-run Health Department. The Mandatory government did not assist in funding health services, but it did provide the National Committee with modest grants, a portion of which was earmarked to cover expenditures on health services in the schools provided by Hadassah through its School Hygiene Department.[65]

While the School Hygiene Department was autonomous in operation and not dependent on the Mandatory Government Health Department, it tended to work with the latter and coordinate matters with Mandatory officials. Their respective directors conducted negotiations between the two bodies, usually by written correspondence. Discussion of matters of principle was carried out by an exchange of letters with Henrietta Szold, in consultation with the director of the School Hygiene Department. The relationship between the two departments had its ups and downs, characterized by disputes over finances and delegation of authority.

Examination of one particular event can illuminate the nature of ties between the two departments and the kind of relationship that existed between them: In 1924, Dr. Berachiahu established a fruitful working relationship with Dr. Raphael Oplatka,[66] a physician employed by the Mandatory Health Department, who was responsible for schools. According to the agreement established between the two doctors, all cases of communicable disease such as typhus, dysentery, diphtheria, and so forth diagnosed among school children and teachers were routinely reported to Dr. Berachiahu. The School Hygiene Department ensured that infected pupils and teachers would remain away from school until cured and until the individual received permission to return. Concurrently, Dr. Berachiahu committed himself to report to Dr. Oplatka all cases of communicative diseases diagnosed by physicians on his staff. This arrangement operated for two years much to the satisfaction of Dr. Berachiahu, who commented: "It signifies that that government Health Department stands behind us...."[67]

This arrangement, however, was altered after Dr. Oplatka was transferred from his post and Dr. Alexander Malchi — a physician from Hadassah Hospital — assumed responsibility for the Communicable Diseases Department of the Government Health Office. Dr. Malchi began carrying out visits to schools on his own, without informing Dr. Berachiahu, completely ignoring the School Hygiene Department and the Educational Department of the National Committee. This move generated bad feelings among personnel in the two departments and among school principals. They complained about the situation to the Education Department. The head of the Education Department in turn broached the issue with government officials, demanding pedagogical issues be referred to the Education Department and matters of hygiene to the School Hygiene Department. Dr. Berachiahu complained to Hadassah management that Dr. Malchi "was derelict in transmission of data and sometimes sent instructions directly to schools, not through our channels."[68] As a result of the complaints, and in keeping with Dr. Berachiahu's suggestion, a new arrangement was inaugurated in 1926, whereby "the government would send instructions regarding education to the Education Department and medical matters regarding schools would be addressed to the Hygiene Department. From this point on, the situation improved."[69] However, it didn't last for long.

Three years later, Dr. Berachiahu again complained, "Now there is no connection between the School Hygiene Department and the Government Health Office."[70] Dr. Chaim Yasski,[71] deputy medical director of Hadassah, intervened in the matter, turning to the Government Health Department, which promised "to improve the situation."[72] In contradiction with its own assurances, however, severance of communication with the School Hygiene Department was carefully preserved. Another three years later,

British authorities published new ordinances that stipulated that "the government will not recognize the directors of the Hygiene and Education Departments, and where necessary, will approach each school directly, both in matters of hygiene and pedagogy."[73]

The Government Health Department did not cooperate with the School Hygiene Department, nor did it contribute to the School Hygiene Department's general budget, arguing that the level of health services enjoyed by the Yishuv in Eretz Israel was a lot higher than that of the Arab community. Therefore, British Mandate policy was to first raise the level of health services for the Arab population, and only afterwards would there be time to address assistance to broaden health services in the Yishuv.

The School Hygiene Department suffered from chronic financing problems. The needs of the Department grew from year to year, while budgets gradually shrank. Dr. Berachiahu was forced to take steps to improve the situation by seeking additional sources of funding. To do so, he turned to the Education Department, informing them of his intention to approach the Government Health Department with a demand to at least "participate in expenditures to cure trachoma in the schools."[74] Dr. Berachiahu attached a detailed statistical report that included the number of treatments administered by his Department in 1928, detailing treatment costs in schools in the cities of Jerusalem, Tel Aviv, Haifa and Tiberias.

The following is some of the information detailing ophthalmologic care administered to school children in Jerusalem, covered in the report — data that illustrates the scope of the work of the School Hygiene Department within the framework of its war on trachoma:[75] ophthalmologic treatments, 597,865; students checked, 8,112; monthly checkups, 3,561; semester checkups, 17,268. The cost of each treatment, including the nurse or doctor's time and medication: 3.07 mil (0.3 Eretz Israel pounds).

Dr. Chaim Yasski, deputy medical director of Hadassah, and Dr. Reuven Katzenelson,[76] deputy director general of Hadassah, approached the Zionist Executive's Secretariat for Health Matters and Henrietta Szold requesting that they support Dr. Berachiahu's request. In their letter, the two praised the important and intensive work of Hadassah's School Hygiene Department over the past decade and the ongoing struggle carried out by the Department against contagious diseases among Jewish school children, through daily systematic examinations by specialists. The two detailed the scope of the Department's work, which encompassed approximately 25,000 pupils under the Department's supervision. Among them, the number of children infected with trachoma reached 10% — that is to say, some 2,500 pupils. The annual Hadassah budget for this purpose was only 5,424 Eretz Israel pounds. Accordingly, Dr. Yasski and Dr. Katzenelson called upon the Government Health Department to take upon itself the funding of this activity because:

> It appears to us that the war on contagious ophthalmologic diseases in Eretz Israel is one of the roles of the Government Health Department, and this demand is totally justified that the Health Department take responsibility for contagious ophthalmologic diseases in Jewish schools.[77]

> Or, they requested, the government should at least "contribute a share in Hadas0sah's budget for this war, by some sum — proportional to what it expends on such activity in government-run schools."[78]

Did the Government Health Department indeed participate in costs of curing ophthalmologic diseases, thus easing the budget of the School Hygiene Department?

The answer lies in the protocols of the "Committee for Investigation of Operative Avenues for the Hygiene Department" that was convened in January 1931, twelve years after the establishment of the Department. Professor Israel Kligler,[79] founder of the Hygiene and Bacteriology Department at the Hebrew University in Jerusalem, who was appointed chairman of the committee, claimed he had learned from reading government reports that the government financed health services and sanitation in government schools operating under its auspices. If this was so, argued Professor Kligler, then "the Education Department of the Jewish Agency should demand governmental participation for hygiene work being done in Jewish schools under its auspices."[80]

Dr. Yasski reported to members of the committee that he had already approached the government about this two years prior, calling upon them to participate "if not totally in our work in the schools, then at least to participate in curing ophthalmologic diseases," noting that "we figured out how much this cost us and turned to the government but it refused."[81]

Dr. Yasski asked Dr. Yitzhak Dov-Berkson, director of the Education Department and a member of the committee, to report whether the government's budget to the Education Department included sums earmarked for hygiene work. Dr. Berkson submitted details of government participation in educational affairs, but explained there was no funding earmarked for hygiene work. He suggested "tying the Hygiene Department's budget to the education budget."[82]

In the end, the Mandatory government did not participate in expenditures on curing ophthalmologic diseases. Hadassah carried all outlays and even continued to underwrite the Department's budget. Indicative of the burden thus imposed, in January 1932 Dr. Yasski sent the School Hygiene budget for the war on trachoma from 1931 to Dr. Berachiahu, requesting:

> *Try to keep within the boundaries of the budget, and even to cut amounts set aside in the budget. We believe it is unnecessary to explain to you just how great the efforts of Hadassah women in America are, in order to find this budget for us and just how much this demands of us under present circumstances — to try and pinch and save as greatly as possible. Only with your assistance — you and all your employees — can we overcome these difficulties.*[83]

After Dr. Berachiahu's failure to receive monitory support from the Mandatory Health Department, with no other option, he turned to the parents of the students and levied a "health tax" of 120 mils[84] per year on each pupil. Dr. Katzenelson, the deputy director general of Hadassah, not only supported the proposal, he even suggested appointing the Education Department to collect the fees. Besides the tax paid by parents, schools were asked to pay 1 Eretz Israel pound per month for the medical work of the School Hygiene Department on their premises — to cover the work of the doctor and nurse and ophthalmologists and dermatologists. Principals tried to avoid payment claiming that the arduous economic straits of the students made this impossible, but Dr. Yasski stood firm that "medical work was so expensive that each school must contribute at least part of the costs."[85]

In this manner — collection of fees from parents and school principals — Dr. Berachiahu succeeded in overcoming financial crisis and balanced the budget of his Department; however, he failed, time after time, in his attempts to achieve a cooperative relationship with the Mandatory government's Health Department, or to receive governmental assistance or financial support for hygiene activities among school children.

The Hygiene Department, the Education Committee and the Education Department[86]

In 1918 a delegation from the Zionist Executive, headed by Dr. Chaim Weizmann, arrived in the country in order to assist the Yishuv and act as a liaison vis-à-vis the military government. The delegation took upon itself responsibility for Jewish education and its funding. During the first year of operation, the Zionist Executive budgeted a large sum to education — a move that contributed to the flowering of education. The Executive established an Education Department under its auspices and equipped it with a larger budget than other departments. But in time, the sizable budget was eroded by the influx of many new students. Jewish education, while suffering from financial and administrative problems, did not enjoy any financial support from the Mandatory government. In 1922, the Mandatory government budgeted a sum of 200 mils per capita (the equivalent of 0.2 Eretz Israel pounds), but this nominal sum was insufficient to cover budget deficits.[87]

In 1922, the Federation of Labor established a Central Cultural Committee that incorporated all the schools and kindergartens in agricultural settlements (15 settlements with a total of 153 children). This network of schools constituted an organizational unit within the Education Department — with almost autonomous administration by the Federation and colored by a clear political bent.[88] Throughout the Mandate period, these schools operating under the auspices of the Central Cultural Committee enjoyed financial support from the Education Department on a group basis, and funding from other sources. Alongside regular schools and the socialist-oriented "workers' network,"[89] a network of ultra-orthodox schools also existed — outside the Zionist camp, encompassing a network of educational institutions, including existing traditional religious schools (Talmud Torah schools) and new religious schools,[90] the latter encompassing secular subjects as well.

How did the School Hygiene Department fit into and operate within the complex educational framework described above? What was the nature of the connection between the Education Committee and the Zionist Executive's Education Department?

The work of the School Hygiene Department was concentrated only in schools within the school network of the Zionist Executive's Education Committee, while schools belonging to the General Federation of Labor's school network were covered by Kupat Holim operations in health matters. Moreover, Kupat Holim forbade doctors and nurses from the School Hygiene Department from entering schools belonging to the workers' network — schools that were under health supervision of Kupat Holim.[91]

Throughout his service as director of the School Hygiene Department, Dr. Berachiahu fought to extend the health services of his Department to encompass all Jewish children and all educational institutions in the country — religious and secular alike. He carried on a mammoth running correspondence with Hadassah on this matter.

In August 1928, Dr. Berachiahu reported to Hadassah management that government doctors practicing in the agricultural townships (*moshavot*) had received permission of the Government Health Office to supervise sanitation in township schools. But in Dr. Berachiahu's eyes, this requirement was not far-reaching enough: The same arrangement should be instituted for doctors working in schools in the city — particularly in regard to ultra-orthodox Talmud Torah schools where there was no supervision whatsoever by governmental health authorities "although bathrooms and water supplies can serve as an important source for spread of contagious diseases."[92] Dr. Berachiahu complained about the phenomenon of total lack of supervision of hygiene and sanitation among Talmud Torahs. He warned that the dire situation was liable to worsen, if the Government Health Office did not take responsibility for supervising the School Hygiene Department of Hadassah, which he headed, because "only in this way can I have hopes of rectifying the sanitary situation in these educational institutions that the government is accustomed to viewing with apathy."[93]

The School Hygiene Department sought to work in cooperation with the Education Committee and the Education Department. Negotiations were conducted between the directors of each body. Reports on organization of the School Hygiene Department — its management and operations — were relayed on a regular basis to the director of the Education Committee. A special "Hygiene Committee" was appointed to mediate between the two bodies in cases of disagreement. The committee was composed of doctors from the School Hygiene Department, representatives of the Education Committee and the Mandatory government supervisor of schools.

For example, one of the disputed issues brought before the committee was: Who will be responsible for recording data in "hygiene ledgers" — records designed to document hygiene and sanitation surveys of schools — the Education Committee or the School Hygiene Department? The question was raised in a meeting of the Hygiene Committee in February 1922 in the presence of representatives of both bodies. Henrietta Szold argued that the Education Committee should be responsible for recording data in the ledgers; however, Yosef Ozerkovsky-Azaryahu, the supervisor of elementary schools and representative of the Education Committee in the Hygiene Committee, responded that this was not the role of the Education Committee. This task cost money, he stressed, and "the Education Committee does not have money for this."[94]

From an organizational standpoint of educational administration, the Education Committee was ranked at the top of the managerial hierarchy — just below the Yishuv's supreme representative body, the National Committee. The Education Department was subordinate to the Educational Committee. The School Hygiene Department, while equal in stature to the Education Department, was "subordinate to the management of the Education Department."[95]

Tense relations typified the link between the two departments — Hygiene and Education — despite their common interest in improving the quality of life of school children. Power struggles that more than once undermined the authority of Dr. Berachiahu prompted him to occasionally turn to Hadassah management to request assistance in settling disputes with the Education Department.

The following is a description of one particular professional dispute — one of many that went on for a number of years — that illustrates the essence of acrimonious relations between the two departments:

Dr. Berachiahu called for integration of first aid courses within the curriculum of teaching seminaries. He reasoned that one should not place children in the charge of a person who does not at least know how to administer first aid when necessary.

Despite the importance of the issue, Dr. Berachiahu found himself, much to his surprise, faced with lack of cooperation from the Education Department. The Educational Department rejected his proposal on managerial-organizational grounds, not pedagogic ones, claiming that the seminar curriculum was "too over-laden as it is, and there is no possibility of adding to it."[96]

Dr. Berachiahu did not surrender, and turned to Hadassah management with a request "to awake the Education Department about this."

Dr. Berachiahu did not give in to the refusal of the Education Department and continued to warn about the need to implement a plan.

In a meeting of the Committee to Investigate Operational Avenues for the School Hygiene Department, Dr. Yasski asked Dr. Berachiahu to report on ties between the two departments in regard to teaching hygiene to kindergarten teachers, teachers, and school children, and steps that had been taken to integrate the subject into school curriculums. Dr. Berachiahu reported that in many elementary schools a hygiene course had already been introduced in the general curriculum, taught by the school nurse. He said that Dr. Yosef Luria — head of the Education Committee — had sent a circular to nature (i.e., science) teachers, instructing them to teach a course in hygiene, and this, indeed, had been done. Dr. Berachiahu also reported that in seminaries in Jerusalem and Tel Aviv, he himself had taught a course in General Hygiene — and more than once, since the seminar students' knowledge of physiology was lacking. Under his recommendation, the Education Committee agreed to introduce this subject into the curriculum as well. Seminar students in Jerusalem even took a course in "First Aid" taught in the hospital. Dr. Berachiahu even suggested the Education Department require all first and second grade teachers to learn first aid, but in his report before the Committee to Investigate Operational Avenues for the School Hygiene Department, Dr. Berachiahu clarified that he had yet to succeed in enforcing this requirement.

The School Hygiene Department worked side by side with the Education Department of the Zionist Executive and tried to function in complete cooperation with it. When Dr. Berachiahu was asked by the Committee to Investigate Operational Avenues for the School Hygiene Department about his ties to the Education Department, he replied:

> *There is a big difference between schools associated with the Education Department and those that are not associated with the Education Department. The better ties are with Education Department institutions. In all matters of sanitation, we turn to the Education Department and it tries to rectify things, as much as feasible.*[97]

The two departments — Education and Hygiene — each had their own budget, planned by their respective directors, but the director of the School Hygiene Department had to channel the reports of his Department through the director of the Education Department. This hierarchical arrangement was not to the liking of Dr. Berachiahu, who denounced overlapping and demanded incorporation of the departments based on the following rationale: The School Hygiene Department and the Education Department deal with

> *The same object in educating the child to a healthy body, spirit and mind to prepare him for life's battles. Moreover, their work is intertwined and tied to one another and cannot be separated. Experience had proven that as long as the two departments were separate authorities with separate budgets, the School Hygiene Department would be merely an advisory organization to the Education Department, its successes would be incomplete, and at times our efforts would be in vain.*[98]

While the School Hygiene Department constituted an integral part of the Education Department, its employees viewed themselves as a separate authority. As an example of such, Dr. Berachiahu cited a grave incident that had taken place in one particular Tel Aviv school: Three janitors were found to be carriers of dysentery germs. He demanded they be immediately banished from the school and not be allowed to be employed as janitors in any educational institution. The Education Department, however, did not accept his recommendation and referred the question to the Health Department of the National Committee. The committee read the report and also recommended that the three be fired immediately. Despite both these recommendations, the three janitors continued work as usual. Dr. Berachiahu complained to Hadassah management that

> *Something like this would not have happened had the director of the Hygiene Department, instead of being a delegate of another department, been a member of the Education Department. This was not an isolated case, and there were many similar cases. School principals do not have the internal authority to fire people in keeping with the demands of another Department. When the Hygiene Department is not an integral part of the Education Department, it cannot protect thousands of school children, open to infection.* [99]

According to the demands of the School Hygiene Department, teachers were required to undergo a general checkup once every two years, but Dr. Berachiahu discovered that many teachers evaded this duty and the Education Department ignored this and did not take serious action against them. Dr. Berachiahu warned against these phenomena "particularly those [who dodge checkup] are the most suspect of having diseases." He accused the Education Department and not the teachers, because they were loyal to the Education Department, and he noted that "a functionary cannot be subservient to two entities." In Dr. Berachiahu's evaluation, only when "the Hygiene Department will not be part of a foreign authority, but rather part of the Education Department, such things will not occur." [100]

With the establishment of the School Hygiene Department, at a meeting of the Committee for Curriculum Preparation, Dr. Berachiahu called for requiring teachers to receive instruction in psychology and hygiene, so they could teach these subjects to their students. For many years, however, he was unsuccessful in realizing this plan. He blamed the Education Department.

Where people sit who are preoccupied with their own demands. The teachers refuse to teach psychology and hygiene, and no plan will be effective as long as there is no professional supervisor of the subject appointed by the Education Department who has the right and the duty to make demands of the teacher and give the order. These things can be actualized only if the Education Department will embody hygiene work within it, as an integral part [of its functions].[101]

Dr. Berachiahu complained that his Department served merely as an advisory body alone to the Education Department, without the authority to fire teachers or janitors who were not suitable for their posts, or to close a school that did not meet sanitary standards set by his Department. He approached Szold in her capacity as head of the Zionist Executive's Education and Health Department, urging her to take action to convince the government to give school physicians the authority to report to the government on deficiencies they encountered in the schools because "if reporting will be the duty of the school physician, it will be easier for us to influence the school administration to carry out our instructions."[102] Dr. Berachiahu even turned to Hadassah management, requesting they take action in favor of incorporation of the two departments, Education and Hygiene, "into one entity, because every day there are problems that require unified work."[103]

Dr. Berachiahu not only requested the consent of Hadassah management to incorporate the two departments, but also even submitted a plan of action, requesting Hadassah's permission to carry it out. According to his plan, funding received from Hadassah, the Mandatory government and the Yishuv would be given to the Education Department

With clear stipulation that these funds would not be used, except for the needs of the Hygiene Department... The Hygiene Department would be subservient to the management of the Education Department. The director of the Hygiene Department — with the aid of the department's physicians — would supervise classroom furnishing, water supply, etc., physical education, the work of the janitor, study of anatomy and personal hygiene in the school. They would have the same authority regarding these subjects as the rest of the supervisor's vis-à-vis their pedagogic subjects.

When the general budget of the Education Department was drawn up, hygiene necessities — such as the work of a nurse and doctor — would be included as an integral part of the Department's operating budget. The governing committee would examine the budget and after approval would monitor the budget [to ensure] it would be spent according to the program approved in advance.[104]

A month after sending this memorandum, Dr. Berachiahu again wrote Hadassah management requesting to add that he had met with Professor Turner, director of the Health Education Department in Boston, who told him that the arrangement he had proposed be applied in Eretz Israel was identical to the order of things in most American cities. At a gathering of experts in health education that had convened in America, it was decided that "this is the best way to educate the young generation in health and a hygienic life."[105]

After twelve years of operation of the School Hygiene Department, Dr. Yasski appointed a special commission headed by Professor Israel Kligler to examine the work of the Department. Professor Kligler, a member of the advisory committee attached to the Straus Health House's Hygiene Guidance Department in Jerusalem, was asked to review the scope of the School Hygiene Department's activities, its operation methods, budget and future development. Dr. Yasski informed Dr. Berachiahu of this, clarifying the commission's mandate.[106]

On the January 3, 1932, the commission convened in the offices of the head of Hadassah. Present were Professor Israel Kligler, committee chairman; Dr. Yitzhak-Dov Berkson, director of the Education Department; Dr. Theodore Zlocisti, a pediatrician with the WIZO (Women's International Zionist Organization) Mother & Child Health Center in Tel Aviv; Dr. Ernst Levi, director of the Public Health Education Department at the Straus Health House in Jerusalem; Dr. Chaim Yasski, director of Hadassah; and Dr. Berachiahu.

In his opening remarks, Dr. Yasski presented the aims of the commission as being "[t]o examine the School Hygiene Department's operational methods based on many years of experience, and to advise it — whether complete changes should be made or alterations introduced in its work and administrative arrangements."[107]

Among other things, the commission dealt with the tie between the School Hygiene Department, the Zionist Executive's Education Department, and the Mandatory government's Education Department. Dr. Berachiahu detailed steps that had been taken by his Department to maintain ties and collaboration with the Zionist Executive's Education Department. He contrasted this with his lack of success in maintaining a normal and productive relationship with the Mandatory government's Education and Health Departments — the latter having refused to even budget for the School Hygiene Department, despite the comprehensive hygiene work it executed in the Jewish school network.

The commission approved Dr. Berachiahu's requests and passed an important resolution that granted Dr. Berachiahu broad authority to operate as an equal, in partnership with the director of the Education Department. Dr. Berachiahu summarized their decision, stating that:[108]

1. Teachers must undergo biannual checkups by a school physician.

2. A teacher who is found to have a health problem will be required to be examined more often, according to doctor's orders.

3. A teacher is not entitled to a post in the Education Department, unless the school physician has first examined him.

4. The Education Department requires teachers to take a course in hygiene. The director of the School Hygiene Department has the right to visit schools, and in the presence of the Education Department supervisor, test students in hygiene.

5. The Education Department will budget annually a sum for repair of furnishings, bathrooms, etc., and will carry out repairs after consulting with the School Hygiene Department.

6. Kindergarten teachers must undergo a course on treatment of children infected with ringworm.

7. Children will not be released from school until they have first been examined by the school physician, who will authorize release (i.e., suspension) — together with the school supervisor.

8. The Education Department will take care of improving the work conditions of janitors.

In August 1932, representatives of the Health Department and representatives of the School Hygiene Department met and gave final approval to additional subjects on the agenda that served as a base for cooperation between the two departments: the Janitors Ordinance; the Teachers' Illness Ordinance; a curriculum for teaching hygiene in elementary schools and teaching seminaries; and a hygiene course for teachers. The decisions passed at this meeting were enforced by employees of both departments — marking the beginning of a new era of cooperation between the two bodies.

The School Hygiene Department and Kupat Holim

The School Hygiene Department operated only in schools run under the auspices of the Zionist Executive's Education Committee, while educational institutions that operated under the auspices of the Cultural Committee of the General Federation of Labor were included in the work program of the General Sick Fund —Kupat Holim. The drawing of separate domains was the result of a power struggle between Hadassah and Kupat Holim that stretched all the way back to when the Unit arrived in the country and worked side by side with Kupat Holim to provide health services to the Yishuv. The power struggles and harsh disputes that arose between the two bodies were primarily over money and control of the medical system in Eretz Israel. As a result, Kupat Holim opposed giving Hadassah doctors the right to enter Federation of Labor–run educational facilities to examine children. Dr. Berachiahu was aware of this problem and was extremely angry because he knew Kupat Holim was prompted by "purely political motivations,"[109] and in his mind, matters of party ideology should not be mixed with health matters.

In light of the ongoing conflicts between Hadassah and Kupat Holim, it is clear why Kupat Holim forbade the School Hygiene Department from operating within schools belonging to the Federation of Labor's Cultural Committee. There were, however, a few special exceptions that were approved in a decision made at a special meeting held in December 1923.

At this meeting, attended by delegates from Hadassah, Kupat Holim and the Federation of Labor's Cultural Committee, deliberations focused on problems existing in Cultural Committee schools that received medical services from the government through Kupat Holim. At the same time, medical and hygiene education activities in Education Committee schools were carried out on an orderly and regular basis by the School Hygiene Department of Hadassah. In the meeting, proposals were made regarding ways Hadassah could rectify the situation and provide the necessary medical assistance to "a number of schools run by the Cultural Committee." Hadassah gave its consent in principle to provide medical services to these schools by its specialists — particularly in the fields of ophthalmologic diseases, dermatology and general hygiene — under the condition that Kupat Holim volunteer "its own personnel" to be responsible for carrying out the orders of the specialists. Consequently, the following decisions were passed:[110]

Nachalat Yehuda: Hadassah doctors would visit the school, and Kupat Holim personnel would carry out their orders. Hadassah would also cover transportation costs; *Rechovot*: Hadassah doctors would visit schools and Hadassah would cover transportation costs; *Shivat Zion* (near Rishon Le Zion): Hadassah doctors would visit the school for Yemenite children. Since Kupat Holim did not have a nurse there, Hadassah would provide a school nurse and pay her salary. Medication would be provided by Kupat Holim from its pharmacy in Nachlat Yehuda.; *Ein Chai, Kfar Saba and Ra'anana*: A Hadassah doctor would carry out the orders of the specialists and in order to reduce travel expenses, the doctors would be transported by the Ein Chai wagon that made frequent trips to Jaffa; *Tel Aviv*: Hadassah doctors would visit the schools populated by the children of labor activists, and Hadassah school nurses working in Education Committee schools would carry out the doctors' orders and provide necessary medical aid.

Dr. Berachiahu was very troubled by the absence of ties between schools associated with the Cultural Committee and those associated with Kupat Holim and the School Hygiene Department. Dr. Berachiahu sought ways to cooperate. He sent numerous correspondences to Hadassah management requesting that they assist him in finding ways to bridge the gap. For example, in March 1931 Dr. Berachiahu sent a memorandum in which he stressed the lack of contact and cooperation between Cultural

Committee schools and the School Hygiene Department under his management. The director asked Hadassah management to intervene and help him find ways to work cooperatively:

> *Until now, there have been no ties for supervision and consultation between the Department and these educational institutions, despite the fact that teachers at these schools have approached us on this matter…More than once I have found Cultural Committee schools that I happened to check by chance, were infected with ringworm — a contagious disease that we have uprooted from our schools…I suggest that Hadassah management find a way to work in collaboration with these institutions.* [111]

Two months later, Dr. Berachiahu wrote Hadassah management again about the same matter, complaining:

> *For eight years, Kupat Holim has not given the Hygiene Department permission to check children in Cultural Committee schools, although the principals and teachers have repeatedly requested our assistance… In that opposition to collaboration is aimed not at the Department and its employees, but against Hadassah for purely political reasons, I think that Hadassah as an apolitical Federation must take the necessary steps in the direction of cooperation.* [112]

Four years later — fifteen years after the establishment of the School Hygiene Department — Dr. Berachiahu was still involved in settling this matter. In February 1935 he sent a letter to Hadassah management reporting that according to his request, Dr. Fritz Noak (Noach), head of the Health Department of the National Council, had approached Dr. Hadassah Heinrich, a leading school physician, suggesting they work together to cultivate a "cooperative program and centralized supervision of all educational institutions in the country."[113] Dr. Noak "treated the appeal sympathetically," for he understood that 2,000 pupils studying in educational institutions of the Cultural Committee should not be isolated and prevented from receiving health services that for over fifteen years had been given to all other children in the country through the School Hygiene Department. Dr. Heinrich accepted Dr. Berachiahu's suggestion but Dr. Tova Berman — a pediatrician destined to be appointed medical director of the Kupat Holim at a later juncture — refused to approve the meeting and forbade Dr. Heinrich from participating. Nevertheless, a month later a work session was held in which Dr. Noak, Dr. Berachiahu and Dr. Heinrich were present. In this meeting the scope of medical and hygiene education work in the schools and ways to incorporate it in all schools was discussed and the following conclusions and decisions were made:[114]

1. There must be cooperation between the work of the school physician of Education Committee schools (Hadassah doctors) and the school physicians of Cultural Committee schools (Kupat Holim doctors).

2. Doctors from both sectors would correlate work methods and maintain direct and ongoing contact between them.

3. The "contracts" drawn up in each sector would be examined by their directors before being sent out. Dr. Berachiahu would hand over the contracts to Dr. Heinrich and Dr. Noak, giving them an opportunity to express their opinion, and they would act in a similar manner.

4. A uniform Pupil's Health Sheet would be employed in all schools.

5. A central archive for storing Pupil Health Sheets would be established in Jerusalem.

6. Dr. Berachiahu and Dr. Heinrich would conduct visits to various schools together, in order to familiarize themselves with the work of each other's sector and formulate a uniform examination method.

7. Joint instructions would be written for all schools regarding the war on contagious diseases.

8. A uniform program would be transferred to all educational institutions in the country regarding diphtheria shots to ensure regularity and accuracy in the future.

9. The war on trachoma would continue and would encompass all schools in the country.

10. The [personal] questionnaire on each child's development that was passed on by kindergartens to elementary schools would be introduced in all kindergartens in the country.

11. Various subjects such as training of doctors and nurses working in schools, hygiene education for students, work in various kinds of schools (Education Department schools, Cultural Committee schools, Mizrachi schools, Alliance schools, private schools and kindergartens), summer camps and other matters would be discussed as needed.

Indeed, following this joint meeting and the decisions reached among the parties, for the first time a professional commission was convened in June 1935 composed of physicians from Hadassah and Kupat Holim. At this meeting it was decided to choose three joint sub-committees — the first to deal with school hygiene, the second to discuss infant care and the third to address treatment of pregnant women.[115]

In this manner — after fifteen years of ceaseless efforts to bring about collaboration and mutual understanding — Dr. Berachiahu finally achieved his goal: an agreement with Kupat Holim that allowed collaboration and uniform work norms on health matters within all schools in the country. Cooperation between the two bodies, as a result of his undying efforts and dogged persistence, constituted a milestone and positive step for the welfare of children and mothers in Israel.

B. Politics and Policy

From the beginning, the School Hygiene Department was directed by Dr. Berachiahu with a strong hand, adopting a strict and unyielding approach based on a centralist policy, opposing any and all intervention by Hadassah management in the workings of his Department or changes in its organization or setup. He was particularly opposed to any intervention by Department physicians in his management style, and more than once expressed himself sharply and with marked cynicism — even outright scorn — regarding Hadassah personnel when he suspected that they were making decisions without consulting him first. Sentences such as, "If I asked not to intrude on my directing the Department as I planned, my intentions were clear,"[116] or, "The work roster in the schools hinges on me and not Dr. Rubinow,"[117] can be found among his correspondence and testify to the director's centralist orientation and dogged and aggressive management style.

Dr. Berachiahu was responsible for all medical, hygienic and sanitation work within the confines of educational institutions in the country that operated under the auspices of the Education Committee.

His post encompassed the following tasks:[118] budget planning and Department expenditures; management of Department ties with government bodies for performance of Department missions; management of ties between the Department and medical teams (school physicians and nurses); setting work conditions of medical teams; general checkups for students at teaching seminary for kindergarten and schoolteachers in Jerusalem and Tel Aviv; management of stations for hard-to-educate children in Jerusalem and Tel Aviv; teaching of courses in spiritual hygiene to school nurses in Jerusalem and Tel Aviv; organization of in-service training seminars for nurses, and guidance and supervision of their work; writing of hygiene course curriculums for elementary schools and teaching seminars; medical checkups for teaching personnel and janitors; and organization of meetings, conferences and national conventions.

How were these tasks and the work of the Department in general reflected in practice? Evidence of the challenges and temper of the times can be gleaned from archival material surrounding one particular gathering of professionals associated with child health issues: a national convention of school physicians held in Jerusalem on April 1, 1928.[119]

The gathering was dedicated to one of the most vexing individual health problems facing the Department — eyesight and trachoma — as well as less focused health issues associated with the physical and mental status of school children in the country and the school environment.

Dr. Berachiahu turned to a number of physicians and requested that they deliver lectures on their areas of expertise. Among those approached were Dr. Yehudit Kozlova, an ophthalmologist who lectured on "Sources of Infection of Trachoma and Ways of Fighting It"; Dr. Ephraim Sinai, an ophthalmologist who lectured on "The State of Trachoma in the Agricultural Township Schools (*Moshavot*)"; Dr. Emanuel Simon, head of the Physical Training Department at the Straus Health House in Jerusalem who lectured on "Physical Treatment in the Schools"; and Dr. Heinz Hermann, a psychiatrist who lectured on "Defective and Psychotic Children in Israel."

Berachiahu was aware of the ramshackle state of many schools — structures in many cases were not suitable to serve as educational facilities. Consequently, he approached Fritz (Peretz) Kornburg, an architect, inviting him to the doctors' convention, requesting that he lecture the gathering on "The Modern School Building in Israel from the Viewpoint of the Architect." Because of the importance of the subject, Dr. Berachiahu sent an invitation to the Association of Engineers and Architects' Jerusalem branch "to take part in debate over this important issue."[120]

Hadassah management, which understood the importance of the convention and its contribution to all those engaged in public health, provided organizational assistance. Dr. Ephraim Bluestone, director of Hadassah, even sent an announcement to physicians and nurses in public medicine departments in Tel Aviv, Haifa, Tiberias, Safed and Jerusalem and approved their participation in the convention "under the condition that the work of the Department or the [physician's] settlement will not suffer on account of this and all the necessary arrangements will be made for a substitute (at no additional expense). The absence of attendees will not come off their annual leave. Travel expenses, of course, will be at their own expense."[121]

The convention was announced and invitations sent to doctors, nurses, educators, the Government Health Department and even the press. Henrietta Szold represented the Zionist Executive; the Education Department sent a delegate of its own, Dr. Yosef Ozerkovsky-Azaryahu. The doctors' convention even found expression in the media of the day: the Hebrew daily *Haaretz* reported the school physicians' convention (March 26, 1928) and *Yidiot Hadassah* printed all the lectures delivered at the conference in a special pamphlet.

Struggles for Control of the Hygiene Department: Chief Nurse Bertha Landsman vs. Dr. Berachiahu

In 1925 Bertha Landsman — head nurse of the infant program of Hadassah in Eretz Israel — was appointed supervisor of all Hadassah public medical institution facilities in the country. In this capacity, she worked side by side with Dr. Berachiahu as the professional responsible for the work of public health nurses.[122] Landsman had received her nurses training at Mount Lebanon Hospital in New York, where many of the head nurses of the Unit had received their training. Upon completion of her studies, Landsman had worked in one of the mother and child stations in New York established by Jewish philanthropist Nathan Straus. In 1921 she immigrated to Eretz Israel. For the first four years, she served as head nurse of infant care stations operated by Hadassah, prior to her appointment as supervisor of all public health nurses.

Within the framework of her new post, Landsman tried to promote a program for hygiene instruction along the lines of similar programs that had been successful in New York. In 1932, when she saw that hygiene studies in various schools were not unified, Landsman submitted a proposal to Dr. Berachiahu and the School Hygiene Department to teach a hygiene and health education course in elementary schools. She claimed that a uniform curriculum was needed. To realize this goal, she suggested the establishment of a special committee comprised of the School Hygiene Department's chief physician; the principal of one of the large schools, chosen by the Education Committee; a teacher from one of the teachers' seminaries; and a school nurse experienced in teaching hygiene. She also suggested what subjects should be encompassed in the curriculum, such as contagious diseases and their prevention, immunizations and disease, and hygiene in the home and personal hygiene. Landsman suggested that this program be taught at the nurses' training school so that all nurses would be able to teach the same curriculum out in the field. Thus, if a nurse or a pupil would transfer schools, the individual would encounter the same subject matter and integrate easily into the curriculum.

In the hierarchy of authority, the chief nurse was subject to the authority of the Department's director, like all the other Department nurses.

Landsman, however, claimed that the nurses were under her authority and her management only. Consequently, dispute over delegation of authority caused serious friction between Landsman and Dr. Berachiahu, echoing more than once in the halls of Hadassah management.

In order to solve the conflict, Hadassah director Dr. Bluestone intervened and ruled that:

> The role of the School Hygiene Department management is to prepare budget and carry out the Department's work plan as approved by the [Hadassah] management. At the same time, the Department director holds responsibility for total and personal supervision of the Department's physicians. Of course, all nurses, without exception should help the Department director realize the program, but they are under the supervision of Mrs. Landsman within her role as executive nurse. At the same time, they are under the discipline and orders of local physicians. However, problems of discipline, dismissal, appointments and transfers shall be transmitted by the executive nurse. I hope that the two departments will help one another in such a way that work will be carried out properly void of disruptions.[123]

Dr. Berachiahu, who opposed all intervention in his authority, sent an emphatic letter in reply:

> The work of school nurses is primarily pedagogic-hygienic-medical. This is raw work requiring direct supervision of an expert to scrutinize the work of the school nurses themselves and to mediate between them and the school administration and the teachers, and to help them every time they encounter pitfalls, and the pitfalls are many, because this work in Eretz Israel is still in its infancy and for a host of reasons cannot be a copy of work in another country.[124] This job is done by me.[125]

Berachiahu even emphasized in his reply that he took pains to transfer all Department reports to the chief nurse (Landsman), as well as all decisions made by the Department or in meetings of doctors and nurses, including a copy of each letter sent to all Department nurses "in a way that all work is always within her view."[126]

Landsman, opposed to the manner in which authority was delegated in Dr. Berachiahu's operation scheme, sent a letter to Dr. Yasski — who had replaced Dr. Bluestone as director of Hadassah — requesting that he delineate authority regarding medical supervision between herself and Dr. Berachiahu. After studying the matter, Dr. Yasski sought to put an end to chronic disputes, suggesting to Dr. Berachiahu that he reach a compromise whereby Landsman would present him with a monthly survey including her reservations and comments on medical work carried out in the schools, and Dr. Yasski would discuss the content with her and with the secretary of the Department, as well as ongoing questions of operation.

This, however, did not bring an end to the disputes and clashes between Landsman and Dr. Berachiahu. The rivalry between them continued throughout the period during which both held their posts. Hadassah management tried — unsuccessfully — to be instrumental in establishing at least civil relations between the two, but to no avail. On April 10, 1932, Landsman presented Dr. Yasski with her reservations regarding the functioning of the School Hygiene Department headed by Dr. Berachiahu, proposing a reorganization plan for school nurses working within the School Hygiene Department. The highly detailed document filled twenty-four pages in English, including explicit suggestions about how to alter the Department's work to improve efficiency.

The paper severely criticized current administrative measures set down by Dr. Berachiahu. Landsman closed the declaration by stating that there was a significant difference in outlook between Dr. Berachiahu and herself regarding the essence of hygienic work in the schools, its realization and administration. She clarified that she would be unable to continue in her position as chief nurse, unless Hadassah management would transfer management entirely to her and to the authority of the Health and Welfare Department that she directed under the auspices of the Hadassah Medical Federation;[127] in essence, she had submitted her resignation. However, from the protocols of the School Hygiene Department it became evident that in actuality, she withdrew her ultimatum and continued to work, although quarrels with Dr. Berachiahu continued in the background.

This state of affairs continued until 1933, when Hadassah management decided to define authority in a manner that would leave no ambiguity: Landsman would supervise public nursing services in the schools, side by side with other public health nursing services already in her hands, and Dr. Berachiahu would supervise medical operations, including the appointment of doctors. The rationale: "This arrangement will free his [Dr. Berachiahu's] honor from the bother of various administrative matters in order to devote more time to actual medical matters."[128]

Landsman remained at her post until 1936.

The Medical Staff

School Physicians

From the beginning, the School Hygiene Department promoted contact and collaboration between school physicians and parents. As part of his job, each school physician was responsible for the health of some 3,000–4,000 pupils. To receive an appointment as a school physician, a doctor had to have psychological-pedagogical training. A doctor lacking expertise in eye and skin diseases could be accepted for work in a school, but was required to undergo comprehensive instruction in treating students infected with trachoma and ringworm.[129]

The role of the school physician focused on two areas:

Medical roles: The physician was responsible for the general development of the pupil, against the background of his natural environment — home and school. His task was "to help the child throughout his school days to grow as a useful citizen in society — this is his primary concern."[130] The doctor checked pupils and dealt with those aspects that require treatment where necessary, such as impairments in sitting posture and eyesight, and teeth in need of dental work, referring pupils for treatment. Prior to extended school outings, he performed a thorough examination and approved participation. The doctor was also charged with educating parents about hygienic habits, at parents' meetings and in personal meetings with pupils. He served as a member of the teachers' council and participated in their meetings during discussions regarding problematic students.

Sanitation roles: The physician was responsible for the school building's setting and orderliness. He supervised the state of lavatories and hygienic arrangements, and was responsible for entering data in the School Hygiene Ledger after conducting sanitation inspections of the school premises. The physician supervised the school cafeteria and took part in planning of meals. School physicians in agricultural townships (*moshavot*) were also responsible for monitoring water supply to the school and were required to fill in a form regarding water supply and whether lavatories were up to standard. The Ledger encompassed:

Toilets: Number of children in the school; number of stalls in toilet facilities; construction material of the toilet; whether doors closed firmly; method of ventilation; whether the facility was equipped to prevent entrance of flies; on what system the facilities operated (pit latrine, pails, siphon); and state of cleanliness.

Water Supply: Whether there was central water supply in the village and of what kind; the source of water to school facilities; whether there was supervision of drinking water quality and of what nature; how drinking water was provided (a container, sink or drinking faucets); whether each pupil had his own drinking cup; and the location of drinking water (in the schoolyard or within the school building).[131]

From reading the reports of Dr. M. Borodetzky — one of the doctors in a Tel Aviv school — the scope of activity and responsibility of the school physician can be appreciated:

> *...I check all pupils without exception because many have not been examined in a year, and many more than a year, moreover, scalp and skin diseases are liable to spread and I think it is correct to check everyone. To date, I have completed examinations of all the students in the Boys' School, the Yemenite Talmud Torah, some six hundred school children in the Girls' School and one hundred and fifty pupils at the Tachkemoni School. I am now adding the Alliance School to my rounds. I have encompassed students and their parents within Hadassah clinic, but few have come. I have invited many mothers to give them instructions regarding their daughters' lice, but they carelessly fail to come...I found the pupils at the Yemenite Talmud Torah to be dirty to an unsurpassed*

degree. I talked to the director of the Talmud Torah and requested that one Sabbath he invite Talmud Torah parents and I would come also to tell them about the danger in such sordidness and the importance of cleanliness. [132]

...I am continuing the general checkup at the Boys' School. Little by little I'm settling into the job, and it is starting to interest me. I check the pupils in groups (in the classroom itself) with the teacher present, serving as an assistant. After the examination, I leave the secretary a list of those pupils who according to their health status are in need [of] treatment or special instructions for their parents that they must visit me at the clinic, together with their sons. [133]

...I finished the general checkup at the Boys' School this week, and have begun checking pupils at the Tachkemoni School. As for my work in general, I am happy to pronounce that I am getting more and more involved and it is becoming more and more interesting for me. Checkups are more pleasant than at the Boys' School because here I encounter a better attitude and more interest from the principal and also from the teachers; it's only too bad that the Tachkemoni School building is so unsuitable for a school. Things should be sped up as much as possible, getting on with construction of the new structure. At the end of August and beginning of January I checked all the students infected with skin diseases and [their] hair. A large number were found to have been cured, or at least having improved the state of their health. It's hard to speak of the girl students, because they refuse to cut their hair. [134]

Dr. Borodetzky's reports embody fascinating data that reflects the tremendous scope of the school physician's role in those days. The workload stemmed primarily from the large number of students under each doctor's supervision, and the multiple tasks for which the school physician was responsible. Other than medical checkups of pupils, Dr. Borodetzky maintained contact with parents and teachers, providing guidance and instruction regarding the health of the pupils.

In this time juncture, there were two central schools of thought in Europe regarding organization of the school physician's work: The school doctor should dedicate only part of his time to the school and most of his time to his private practice, or the school doctor should dedicate all of his time to school-related medicine and refrain from engaging in private practice entirely. The first school of thought was the dominant one, but did not produce desired results.

The reason was that school hygiene encompassed so many areas: School doctors had to be knowledgeable about public health, general hygiene, childhood diseases, contagious diseases, psychology, pedagogy and child psychiatrics. A doctor also engaged in private practice was not always free to gain expertise in all of these medical fields. Consequently, school physicians who maintained private practices tended naturally to concentrate most of their time on professional advancement of their own particular area of expertise. Thus, there was a danger that the school physician's work in the school would be neglected in the interest of expanding his private practice.

Dr. Berachiahu, director of the School Hygiene Department, adopted the model of the full-time school physician from the start, following Dr. Rubinow's restrictions on private practice that had been implemented in 1919 as a leading principle of Hadassah activity in Eretz Israel. He ensured that in all locations where there were large educational institutions, the school physician would dedicate all his time to his work in the school system and would not engage in private practice. Indeed, his policy was justified by the evidence in schools where there were only part-time physicians. The performance of the part-time school physicians was found to be lacking in comparison with the work of full-time physicians. More than once, "partial physicians" were replaced by "complete doctors."

One such case in Tel Aviv is instructive: Dr. Vilenchik began to work as a school physician in place of Dr. Schwartz, concurrent with her work at the hospital. Over time, her work in the school was neglected, and Dr. Berachiahu, who reported the situation, sent an angry letter to Dr. Meshulam Levontin, Hadassah branch director in Jaffa, about the work in the school that had been neglected, stating:

> My opinion has always been that two jobs should not be combined, hospital and school together, except under one condition: that the entire morning be devoted to schools. Clearly, then the physician must be endowed with a great deal of energy and ability for working.[135]

Dr. Berachiahu was aware of the fact that the work of a school physician — despite its responsibility — was considered less prestigious than the work of a specialist engaged in private practice or a doctor on hospital staff. In his own estimation he had indicated that "school physicians working a full day without the right to a private practice and without the right to cure [patients] — no doctor who values himself would agree to take on such a post. He would be nothing but a clerk on a lower footing than a public nurse."[136] Therefore, Dr. Berachiahu sent a memorandum to Hadassah management in which he detailed his recommendations regarding employment of school physicians:

A doctor should be appointed for each city, responsible for all hygiene work — medical and administrative — in schools, in the city and its environs. The doctor should be forbidden from engaging in private practice and should devote all his time to this broad-scoped profession that demands ongoing advanced studies to stay abreast.

> A "full time doctor" working in schools is not permitted to engage in private practice. The morning hours will be devoted to work in the school and the afternoon to work in the students' clinic.

> In settlements where there is not full-time work, it is possible to allow private practice only if there is no possibility of employing the physician in other public health work, such as: treatment of infants and toddlers, tuberculosis patients and the deformed in a clinic or hospital. In any case, the doctor should be committed to carry out his part-time position in the school in the morning hours, and limit complimentary work to after-school hours.[137]

In a meeting of school physicians held in Tel Aviv in September 1923, a proposal was raised that school nurses be replaced by fledgling physicians, to allow the doctors to specialize in school hygiene and in this way allow them to supplement their income. Dr. Berachiahu, arguing that doctors would demand higher salaries than nurses:

A nurse receives 7–8 pounds and I think we can't require a doctor to work for such a small sum as this. A fledgling physician that will work daily, six hours straight at this monotonous task will be quickly fed up with it and become contemptuous [of his role] but unable to specialize in other fields of medicine, and after a year and a half will forget all he studied — being neither doctor nor nurse, but rather a holder of a doctor's diploma — an unpleasant state of affairs from a number of standpoints.[138]

Some of the doctors supported Dr. Berachiahu's position and argued "the nurses provide more benefit than a physician."

Dr. Berachiahu concluded the issue, saying:

> A school nurse remains all day in the [educational] institution and acts as a liaison between the parents' home, the school and the physician. She is responsible for all the hygiene work in the school: curing eye and skin diseases, bandages, home visits, weighing, measuring and supervision of cleanliness.[139]

Therefore fledgling physicians should not be introduced "only due to pity for young doctors." He was opposed to replacing nurses with young doctors primarily because "this work is for a nurse and is not suited for a man, even if he is a doctor."

In other words, the School Hygiene Department from its early stages stood firmly behind the necessity of creating a close tie between the physician, the school and the pupil's home. The assumption was that period checkups conducted in the schools were not sufficient for school physicians to monitor the general health status of the pupil and did not allow him to be well acquainted with the pupil. In the framework of his work, the school physician was responsible for some 3,000–4,000 pupils. At times he had to conduct additional checkups to deepen his knowledge about a particular pupil — such as information on sleep and diet patterns; leisure time activities; the pupil's status in the family and so forth; and talks with parents — to explain and advise them and provide suitable care. For this the doctor needed a reception room in a central clinic, "a place where pupils from different institutions can turn, in accordance with the instructions of their teacher, the doctor himself or the nurses."[140] To fulfill this purpose, special clinics for school children were established. The work of the pupils' clinics made it possible for a school physician to engage in curative medicine. This arrangement addressed undercurrents of dissatisfaction in professional circles, as a number of physicians had argued that "a doctor that doesn't treat patients and sees only 'healthy' children in schools, and has no contact with a clinic, cannot develop and is even liable to forget his learning. An enlightened physician would not agree in any way to reduce his scientific endeavors to being satisfied with merely checking pupils in the school."[141]

Experience showed that the number of schoolchildren coming daily to the clinic was 20 to 30 a day — most if not all from low-income families, "in need of constant supervision." It was also shown that every month there was a good number of cases of contagious diseases diagnosed that had it not been for the pupils' clinics would not have come to the attention of school physicians and principals. Thanks to the clinics, it was possible to cure pupils infected with ringworm with Thallium.[142] Such children needed to be closely watched over a period of months including urine tests, weighing and monitoring of hair loss — medical supervision carried out by the clinics.

Dr. Arieh Dostrovsky,[143] chief dermatologist at the Hadassah Medical Federation who also served as a school physician, testified to the effectiveness of the system:

> In no other country has there been such good results in curing ringworm among children as we have had, and the reason is only due to [the fact] that supervision is intensive and for this reason more frequent. The pupil has a center where he must go to receive necessary daily treatment that must not be neglected.[144]

Side by side with the pupils' clinics run by school physicians, special residential infirmaries (batei marpeh) were established in large cities with a large concentration of pupils. The importance of these facilities was tremendous, since at times it was necessary to monitor the health status of the pupil to determine the symptoms of his illness, and at the same time to watch the child to gather information on the state of his health and conditions in the home. The pupil stayed at the infirmaries until diagnosed. In addition, the facilities provided supervision of children suffering from active tuberculosis or malaria until their recovery. Many pupils diagnosed with "enlarged spleens"[145] were hospitalized in residential infirmaries for schoolchildren, receiving intensive care until their full recovery. Dr.

Berachiahu commented that in the clinics "important public health work was done for the growing generation."[146]

Specialists

The School Hygiene Department adopted the outlook that even the first initial checkup of pupils — including eyes, skin, teeth, bones and so forth — should be conducted by a specialist. This was contrary to the prevailing attitudes in European countries where it was felt such checkups should be conducted by a general practitioner, and only if the physician found a child infected with a disease that required treatment by a specialist would parents be advised to send their child to the proper specialist. The School Hygiene Department ensured that eye examinations, dental checkups and an orthopedic examination would be conducted by specialists. Thanks to the various specialists who were employed by Hadassah Hospital, the Department was able not only to grant schoolchildren treatment by specialists, but also their first general checkup. In addition, School Hygiene Department physicians were able to refer pupils to Hadassah's x-ray and bacteriology labs when such a step was necessary to reach a diagnosis.

In early 1927, orthopedic examinations by a school physician were introduced in Jerusalem and Tel Aviv, under the supervision of an orthopedic specialist. For this purpose a special Orthopedic Ledger was drawn up, and doctors and nurses working in schools were required to undergo a special course in orthopedic gymnastics.

School Nurses

School nurses enjoyed Dr. Berachiahu's appreciation from the beginning, due to their dedicated and intensive work in the schools. Dr. Berachiahu expressed this emphatically, noting:

> There isn't a country, not in Europe and not in the United States, that can compare to us in the scope of medical and hygiene education [carried out by] the school nurse, and her broad circle of influence. Besides the tasks common to nurses everywhere, here in Eretz Israel where levels of

personal and general hygiene are on a very low level, the nurse has a very important role as a teacher-educator in practical hygiene in the schools. By home visits, and by doing so disseminating knowledge of daily hygiene while taking upon herself the role of instructing the People on [matters of] practical hygiene.[147]

Posts as school nurses were open only to nurses who had completed their studies at a nursing school and attended nine months of special training in public health work. These nurses worked in schools in the dual role of school nurses and of practical hygiene teachers. At the closing ceremonies of the seventh graduating class of Hadassah's nursing school held on December 6, 1927, the school director, Hadassah Schedrovitzky-Sapir, noted changes in the school curriculum, including the fact that "public [health] work was removed from the regular curriculum of the school and only students endowed with special character [required by] this profession would be allowed to study it."[148]

The work of the school nurse encompassed three areas:

Therapeutics: General checkups of pupils that included measuring and weighing, examination of personal cleanliness, treatment for lice, ringworm and trachoma according to doctor's orders, and administration of immunization inoculations against contagious diseases and first aid. *Educational-Scholarly*: Teaching lessons in public health according to a set program that included instruction in subjects such as personal and general hygiene, instilling orderly and healthy nutrition and care of food; maintenance of proper sleep and an orderly lifestyle; instillation of hygienic habits such as washing hands after use of the toilet and before eating, and use of a clean and personal handkerchief; organization and instruction in Health Fellowships;[149] distribution of cod liver oil and a glass of milk; guidance for parents; home visits; and bimonthly parent meetings together with the school principal, homeroom educator and school physician. These gatherings were devoted to discussion of child hygiene matters — subjects such as nutrition, personal cleanliness, sleep, and child health, and hygienic preservation of foodstuffs.

Sanitation: Supervision of cleanliness and order in the school and supervision of the work of the janitor.

The school nurse was responsible not only for schoolchildren but also for their families. Families were familiar with the school nurse, and she was perceived by parents to be an authoritative source on matters of health and hygiene. Mothers even made her party to private matters such as relations with their spouses, problems in schooling, economic straits, difficulties during pregnancy and so forth. In those days, to a certain extent, the school nurse served as a kind of social worker.

The nurse was the close assistant of the school physician. Dr. Berachiahu stressed that "the work of the school physician without an assisting nurse at his side would be, in our times — impossible. Only in places where there is a public nurse is the value and the influence of the physician evidenced."[150]

The high value he assigned his Department's nurses prompted Dr. Berachiahu to protect their status and rights; contribute to the enhancement of their professional stature; and broaden their education through in-service training and courses in pedagogy and medical pedagogy. He even contacted the management of the National Library in Jerusalem to arrange access for nurses to take out books and magazines, maps and charts from the medical library that were necessary for the work of nurses engaged in public medicine. Likewise, he arranged for lectures at schools and "Health Scout" clubs, and provided guarantees for the safe return of professional literature taken on loan.

Work Conditions

Salaries

The salaries of school nurses amounted to 7 Eretz Israel pounds a month. Yearly, when the Department's budget was being drawn up, the question of nurses' salaries were raised as an avenue for cutting costs. Such was the case when Dr. Berachiahu planned the budget for schools in Jaffa with the help of the District Physician Dr. Menachem Stein. Dr. Stein suggested reducing nurses' salaries to 5 Eretz Israel pounds a month to "ease" the budget. Dr. Berachiahu was opposed, arguing that nurses incur hidden expenses such as "the necessity of coming to school in clean dresses and polished shoes, etc. and one cannot compare her in this matter to a worker on the road or in collective settlements (*kvutzot*)...I would therefore request to inform the nurses that their salaries will be 7 *lirot* [Hebrew plural for pounds]."[151]

In 1931, a proposal was raised by Hadassah management to match salaries of school nurses with those of nurses in hospitals. Dr. Berachiahu rejected this suggestion, arguing that "carrying out of this decision is not justified, for matching salaries will certainly lead to a drop in work standards that we have succeeded in perfecting and bringing to a high level."[152] In a letter to Hadassah management, Dr. Berachiahu described the track for professional advancement of nurses, from graduation from nursing school up until acceptance for a post within the School Hygiene Department:

A nurse completing nursing school is accepted for an advanced studies course. Only those suitable for such are accepted for the extra nine-month course. From among the enrollees, again, only those deemed suitable for work in the schools are chosen. School nurses, therefore, are endowed with knowledge, talents and wisdom that are not found among other nurses. Therefore, they should not be placed on an equal footing.[153]

Alongside the school nurses there were special "skin and eye" nurses that administered medical treatment to pupils afflicted with trachoma and ringworm. These nurses worked under the supervision of the school nurse and their salary amounted to 5.50 Lira a month. In November 1924 "skin and eye" nurses' salaries were upgraded to six Lira a month. Nurses who administered treatment for ophthalmological diseases were under the supervision of ophthalmologists and were accepted for employment in the schools after consultation with Dr. Ticho, chief ophthalmologist at the Hadassah Medical Federation. Nurses that dealt with skin diseases were under the supervision of a dermatologist and were accepted for employment after consultation with Dr. Dostrovsky.

Leave

On March 24, 1926, an agreement was signed with school nurses and "skin and eye" nurses granting them the right to paid annual leave during the Jewish holidays in the fall and Passover in the spring — a total of 22 days of leave. Regarding Sabbath days, school trips and so forth when regular school was not in session, they were committed to work in places where the branch administration sent them, such as "to come to aid in the hospital."[154] This arrangement continued until 1930, and was accompanied by disputes and friction between the School Hygiene Department and the nurses. The Department demanded that during school vacations nurses would assist in hospitals according to the needs of Department branches in their particular city while the nurses requested to utilize the time to catch up on administrative work, update Pupil Health Charts and read professional literature. Dr. Yasski intervened and decided that during school vacations nurses would work half-time in the school, utilizing the time for home visits, and devote the rest of the time to professional literature and administrative tasks.

Conventions and Meetings of School Nurses

Once a year, a National Convention of School Nurses was held at which time professional issues arising at work were debated. For instance, at the Convention held on September 28, 1931, issues such as the hygiene curriculum, organization of work with the Health Fellowships, and suggestions for subjects to discuss at Parents Meetings were addressed.

Once a month, the school physicians and school nurses in each city met jointly to discuss difficulties encountered in their work together and to seek ways to improve and economize. In a joint meeting held in Tel Aviv on June 17, 1929, the following issues were raised:

Dysfunction of janitors in the schools:

The Tel Nordau School nurse complained that the level of cleanliness in the school was extremely low. She specified:

> *Doors and windows are dirty, floors are washed only twice a week and without soap... The janitor promised to clean but has not done so. And this is the situation in other schools as well in which she works. The janitors do not have enough time to clean, and during recesses the female pupils help with cleaning.[155]*

The nurse at the Talpiot School complained that "in the morning the janitor removes dust from the furnishings with a feather duster thus raising dust just before classes." At one of the schools for girls, the nurse reported that "the janitors don't dust at all." Dr. Berachiahu subsequently decided: "Janitors are required to dust with a damp rag half an hour before school starts." He reported his decision to the Educational Department.

Whether to allow boys and girls to sit on the same bench:

It was decided that in coed schools, pupils should be allowed the freedom to choose. In exceptional cases, teachers should supervise and consult with the school physician.

Female hygiene:

Regarding how to teach lessons in female hygiene in coed schools, the decision was to conduct special classes for girls only.

Enrichment courses for school nurses in pedagogy:

Dr. Berachiahu announced that a course in pedagogy for school nurses would be held during the summer.

The school nurses' congested schedule:

The school nurses complained that they worked six hours straight without a break because during recesses, while teachers were able to relax, the school nurses had to treat the children. Dr. Berachiahu suggested cutting the nurse's hours and promised to consult the school principals on the matter.

Weekly meetings of school nurses took place in every city. At these gatherings, subjects common to the city's schools and core questions concerning ongoing work were discussed. One such meeting among school nurses in Tel Aviv discussed, for instance:[156] Organization of distribution of cod liver oil in the school; dental services for Tel Aviv children and who was exempt from payment; dysfunction of janitors; children with learning difficulties and the need to organize a suitable framework for them; and health diaries and whether pupils should be required to keep them.

The nurses worked under the supervision of the School Hygiene Department's director Dr. Berachiahu and chief nurse Bertha Landsman. In each city one nurse was chosen to serve as a supervisory nurse whose job was to oversee the work of all the public nurses in the city, chair staff meetings and maintain ongoing contact with the chief nurse in Jerusalem.

Chana Weissman, supervisory nurse for Tel Aviv, reported to Dr. Berachiahu and to Dr. Yitzhak Alterman — head of the Education Department in the Tel Aviv Municipality — on a decision made during a nurses' meeting to organize a Health Week:[157]

> *A Health Week committee shall be appointed in each school whose members would be comprised of the school principal, a delegate from among the teachers and the school nurse. It was decided to conduct the following activities during Health Week: To organize a thorough cleaning of the school with the participation of the schoolchildren and members of the Health Fellowship; to conduct informative discussions for teaching staff on typhus and dysentery; to organize parents' meetings with doctors, accompanied by an image projector to organize activities among the children including writing essays, slogans and adages and drawing pictures on the theme How to Keep Healthy, and to give prizes for outstanding work; to organize a competition among classes for the cleanest classroom, and to grant a circulating prize for the best classroom; to prepare a play on the subject "The Fly" that would be presented by members of the Health Fellowship before the student body of all schools.*

The broad scope of the school nurse's work endowed her with special status within the school and within the community where she resided and worked. She constituted an authority on all aspects of health and hygiene, serving as a contact for parents, teachers and children alike. Her intensive, efficient and devoted work spurred the expansion and enhancement of health and hygiene activity in educational institutions in the country, raising their standard to a reputable level that was destined to serve as a guiding model for the role of school nurses even after the establishment of the State of Israel in 1948.

C. Areas of Activity of the School Hygiene Department

The School Hygiene Department focused on health and hygiene work in five areas: general medical supervision of pupils and dispensation of ambulatory care; dermatological treatment and follow-up; ophthalmological treatment and follow-up; medical-hygienic treatment and follow-up of pupils, teachers and janitors; and hygienic-sanitary treatment and follow-up of educational institutions.

General Medical Supervision of Pupils and Dispensation of Ambulatory Care

The medical supervision encompassed general physical checkups, orthopedic supervision and physical education, supervision of school outings and examination of their impact on students.

General Physical Checkups

The school physician carried out general physical checkups of pupils twice a year. Schoolchildren found to be infected with a disease were summoned to the Pupils' Health Clinic together with their parents to receive treatment and medication. Each student was weighed, measured, inoculated against tuberculosis, underwent a eyesight and hearing test and from time to time received immunization shots and smallpox vaccinations. This arrangement existed during the first years following establishment of the School Hygiene Department. After the number of students stricken with malaria dropped significantly, the state of trachoma improved, ringworm was entirely eradicated and the hygienic-sanitary status of educational institutions improved, annual physicals were adopted in lieu of twice a year. With the establishment of Pupils' Health Clinics and an increase in the number of school nurses, annual physicals were replaced by physical checkups once every two years.

The school doctor visited schools once a week to check schoolchildren. The school nurse registered checkup results on each pupil's personal Health Chart. Deficiencies found during the checkup — such as lack of cleanliness, poor nutrition, sclerosis and so forth — were recorded on a Deficiency Card that remained with the nurse for follow-up and subsequent checkups. After the pupil recovered, the Deficiency Card was "closed" and attached to the child's Health Chart.

Orthopedic Supervision and Physical Education

At first, physical education did not receive sufficient attention in schools in Israel. In 1856 Dr. Ludwig-August Frankel — an ophthalmologist, poet and writer — arrived in Jerusalem. As general secretary of the Jewish Community in Vienna, Dr. Frankel's goal was to establish a shelter for children named in honor of the aristocratic family Lamel from Prague. His plan was to combine religious studies with secular studies, side by side with teaching the children "to make movements with their bodies to strengthen their character and health."[158]

His intentions aroused fierce opposition among ultra-orthodox (*haredi*) circles in the Yishuv in Jerusalem and its leaders who vehemently opposed this curriculum plan and did everything in their power to prevent establishment of the institution. The ultra-orthodox leaders claimed it was "a worthless thing to strengthen their bodies by gymnastic exercises... Our children do not need to strengthen the body or play outside. Schools where they will learn some other subject in addition to Talmud will lead to throwing off the mantle of religious duties of the Torah and religion."[159] Therefore, they suggested Dr. Frankel abandon his plans and transfer his support to dressing and feeding students in the *heder* (i.e., traditional Jewish elementary educational frameworks).

Despite opposition — including bans, and protest posters on the walls against Dr. Frankel — the Lamel School was opened in 1856, becoming the first school to encompass gymnastics as part of the curriculum program. At the time of construction of a new school building for the school in 1903, Principal Efraim Cohen took care to install gymnastic equipment in the schoolyard as was common in Germany. Special attention was given to developing healthy bodies, and in each class two hours a week were devoted to gymnastics. Moreover, the Lamel School hired a special instructor — Jerusalem-born Avraham-Zvi Goldshmidt who had studied gymnastics in Holland. Goldshmidt was the first professional gymnastics teacher in the country; he also taught at the Girls' School, and was an influential figure in the development of physical education in Israel in general.[160]

On the eve of World War I, gymnastics curriculums underwent a change in development. In 1913, the various Gymnastics Associations in Eretz Israel merged into one federation with nine branches. The Association engaged in sport, hiking trips, processions and games.[161] While gymnastics were introduced into the curriculum in a portion of the schools, other schools entirely ignored the subject — particularly religious educational institutions.[162] Gymnastics were not considered a genuine subject worthy of a formal place in a school curriculum, and the physical development of children was still not recognized as important. Consequently, in physical checkups conducted by school physicians under the auspices of the School Hygiene Department, a significant percentage of children was found to be suffering from skeletal deficiencies.

In Jerusalem Dr. Emanuel Simon, head of the Orthopedic Gymnastics Department of the Straus Health House, conducted checkups. Among 11,000 pupils, the following deficiencies were found: lordosis (concave back), 2.0%; kyphosis (rounded back), 4.0%; sclerosis (curvature of the spine), 11.7%; foot defects, 11.3%; poor posture, 25.6% (boys) and 26.5% (girls).[163] In Tel Aviv the situation was worse: Among 2,109 pupils that underwent orthopedic examinations, 375 (22.1%) were found to suffer from poor posture; 672 (39.5%) had sclerosis; and 1,026 (60.4%) had foot defects.[164]

Dr. Berachiahu blamed the Education Department, school principals and teaching faculty, arguing that they neglected physical education and did not take care of the acquisition of suitable furnishings to maintain good posture. Therefore, he demanded:

The number of hours devoted to gymnastics [is] too few, moreover there is not sufficient furniture, and the main thing — there is no supervision of seating of children in the classroom. Correct sitting posture when reading and writing do not exist in our schools. There is no attention to gymnastic and orthopedic care, teachers are not strict about maintaining proper posture among their students. The children enter school in a normal state [with] straight backs but as they proceed toward the upper classes, the number of children with crooked backs increases.[165]

Furthermore, Dr. Berachiahu said that present furnishings in schools were not suitable for the ages and heights of the students:[166]

Sitting [arrangements] are very bad, and the medical personnel have no right to supervise physical education. Except for gymnastics (1–2

hours a week) they lack the ability to rectify what is wrong — 6 hours of
bad sitting posture daily. Students in the Talmud Torahs have been found
to have hunched backs... of the worst kind from sitting on benches, and
there is not gymnastics there at all. ...

In a report sent by Dr. Berachiahu to Hadassah management after
visiting educational facilities in Machane Yehuda, he wrote: "In the Talmud
Torahs children still sit on the floor in a dimly-lit room around one copy
of the Pentateuch, reading from all sides."

Dr. Berachiahu did not have the authority to demand rectification
of the situation without the approval of the Education Department.
The Education Department, however, was in no hurry to cooperate.
Consequently, Dr. Berachiahu turned to Hadassah management. He
reported the results of orthopedic examinations to them, warning:

All the gymnastics teachers and doctors that have worked in schools
abroad are aware of the large number of children here with skeletal
deficiencies. Our children don't know how to sit [or] how to stand, and
there is a large number that don't know how to breathe properly. The
matter should be studied, visits conducted in gymnastics classes and
consultation carried out with gymnastics teachers about additional or
different gymnastic exercises needed by a student — in the school or in
the home, and to follow results.[167]

However, Dr. Berachiahu's main complaint to Hadassah was that as
long as the School Hygiene Department was merely an advisory body to
the Education Department and had no right to directly supervise physical
education, it could not bring about improvement, and "there is no hope
of enhancing the situation."[168] Consequently, Dr. Berachiahu decided to
integrate this important issue in the 2nd Convention of School Physicians
that was held in Jerusalem on April 1, 1928.

In this regard, he approached two orthopedic experts — Dr. Emanuel
Simon and Dr. Ernst Levi — asking them to present lectures on the
subject at the upcoming convention. Dr. Levi lectured on "orthopedic
gymnastics." Dr. Simon spoke about "the necessity of introducing daily
gymnastics lessons in the elementary school curriculum"[169] based on
the findings of his orthopedic examinations of Jerusalem schoolchildren.
In his letter to the Hadassah management, Dr. Berachiahu even asked

Hadassah to consider opening a school to train gymnastics teachers and to appoint a special supervisor of gymnastics curriculums in Israel.

At the 1928 School Physicians' Convention, the doctors passed important resolutions regarding physical education including:

All teachers must take care of the physical safety of their pupils. They must seek to reduce the damage school life inflicts on their students. The means: a. supervision of correct sitting posture in the classroom; b. three-minute breaks for physical exercises in the classroom, in the middle of scholastic lessons; c. games involving physical activity during recess between class periods.

Physical education classes must be held. The duration should be a half hour daily (games and exercises) for the lower grades; every other day (three times a week) for the middle grades; and once every three days (twice a week) for the upper grades.

In order to train teachers to carry out roles as those responsible for the physical development of children, it is necessary to: a. set enough gymnastics lessons in teaching seminaries — for all classes (not less than three a week) in order to train future teachers to conduct gymnastics lessons for children; b. the Education Department must organize summer in-service training for teachers on teaching gymnastic.

School physicians and gymnastic teachers must maintain ongoing contact and plan physical education together.

The Education Department will appoint one general supervisor or district supervisors of physical education in the schools.

A teacher will be appointed principal only after receiving special training in school hygiene and physical education.[170]

In accordance with the decisions made at the Convention, Dr. Berachiahu sent the Education Department's school supervisors directives on body hygiene, stipulating that one should take care to maintain proper posture among students while reading, writing and listening by: a. conducting two minutes of free exercises in the midst of lessons — about 20–25 minutes from the outset of the lesson; b. measuring the height of students every three moths; c. switching seating arrangements of students sitting at the sides of the classroom, if the blackboard is not hung in the middle.[171]

Dr. Berachiahu did more than just talk — he also took personal action. The students' posture problem bothered him immensely, so he took it upon himself to design a "hygienic chair for students" that would provide stable and comfortable seating, prevent development of skeletal deficiencies, occupy less space in the classroom, "and would be easy to move about"[172] and would be suitable for all the various kinds of work carried out by the student in the class: reading, writing and crafts. The chair, constructed by a furniture factory according to specifications, was placed on display in the Jerusalem Gymnasium and chairs were ordered for the institution in accordance with its proportions.[173]

In order to enhance orthopedic work and encompass a large number of pupils in need of orthopedic treatment, Dr. Berachiahu wrote to Professor Israel Kligler — a member of the advisory committee attached to the Straus Health House's Hygiene Guidance Department — requesting approval of his proposal that gymnastic teachers undergo special training in orthopedic gymnastics to allow them to work out with children in need of this kind of corrective exercise. The schoolchildren would pay according to means and poor pupils would be exempt from payment. Dr. Berachiahu even requested that Professor Kligler approve printing illustrations of "proper and improper posture" to hang on classroom walls. "These illustrations, hung on the walls in front of the pupils will be a reminder of proper posture for both teacher and pupils."[174]

In June 1936, Dr. Berachiahu sent a plan for orthopedic gymnastics in the school to Dr. Yitzhak Alterman, head of the Education and Culture Department in the Tel Aviv Municipality, requesting strict adherence to the plan. According to the plan formulated in the School Hygiene Department, schools should be furnished (i.e., with tables and chairs) according to standards set by the School Hygiene Department and should organize orthopedic gymnastics in the afternoon and make school principals responsible for their execution. The principals would visit lessons from time to time and take measures against those dodging participation. In addition, each teacher would receive from the school nurse a list of those of her students with defective posture in order to supervise the child's posture in the classroom, because "without this kind of supervision, there is no value to orthopedic gymnastics."[175] Furthermore, Dr. Berachiahu ordered school nurses to instruct parents on how to deal with proper posture of their children in the home. In these ways, Dr. Berachiahu hoped to improve the posture of school children in Israel, and rectify existing skeletal deficiencies.

Supervision of School Hiking Trips and Examination of Their Impact on Students

Teachers in Israel viewed hikes as an important educational tool. Among the first teachers to recognize the special value of hiking was Efraim Cohen, who inaugurated this innovation in the Lamel School from the beginning. The rationale: "Short trips in the city and its environs and hikes to distant places for observation purposes is an important aide for learning about the homeland and the Bible, and to strengthen ties with the homeland."[176]

Simcha-Chaim Vilcomintz, a teacher and supervisor of schools in the agricultural townships (*moshavot*) of the Upper Galilee said in a lecture on the curriculum in township schools: "Hikes have been customary in the schools and are beneficial for physical and moral education. Once or twice a month the teachers will take their pupils to one of the cities or agricultural townships, or to one of the nearby villages."[177]

The recognition of hiking as a way to know and become familiar with the land was first addressed in the gymnasium and teachers' seminary in Jerusalem. Their graduates were the first to engage in adult education and organize trips. The emphasis was not just on familiarity with the country, but also on nurturing a new local milieu that included field trips and camping, adopting special clothing, songs and patterns of behavior, and above all, developing a deep tie with the land.[178]

Within his role as head of the School Hygiene Department, Dr. Berachiahu was aware of the educational-national merits of hikes. As a doctor, however, he was also aware of their health value. In order to make school principals more aware of the dangers inherent in hikes, in

February 1928 Dr. Berachiahu sent a circular to school principals updating them on research regarding the effect of hikes on pupils from both a physical and psychological standpoint. The result of his study stressed the fact that "these hikes tire the children too much, and instead of being beneficial they are detrimental."[179] In order to prevent possible damage, Dr. Berachiahu formulated rules "regarding the distance of hikes graduated to age, flat plains and mountains separately."[180]

He ordered school nurses to weigh the pupils and take the measurements of their chests with a spirometer before any extended hike. The nurses were directed to retake measurements and weight immediately upon the pupils' return, and a third time six to seven weeks later. After receiving the results from school nurses, he would analyze the data and provide the schools with the results for use of teachers giving hygiene lessons. In this manner, children would be taught "the effect of an orderly hike according to the rules and the damage that is done by excessive sports exercises that are not conducted under the supervision of an experienced leader who knows how to keep things in proportion."[181]

In order to make principals and teachers aware of the importance of going out on hikes, as well as the health and hygiene perils involved, Dr. Berachiahu wrote memorandums to schools and teachers' seminars in which he outlined "hiking procedures" as follows:

Teachers would inform the School Hygiene Department at least two days prior to any hike. During this time, the school physician would review Pupil Health Charts of all participants and determine whether all could participate, and would prepare medical equipment for them.

There would be special regulations regarding purchase of food: Buying food for trips lasting several days would not be left to the students, but rather one person or more will be appointed to buy for all the hikers and the appointed persons will be responsible [for ensuring] that fruit will be dipped in boiling water two to three minutes before eating. In addition, the hike leaders will be responsible [for ensuring] that hikers will not eat in various eateries without [the establishments] being scrutinized, but rather only in those kept in a clean state.[182]

In the 2nd National Convention of School Physicians held in Jerusalem in April 1928, the subject of hikes and their effect on pupils was also addressed. During Convention deliberations, resolutions were passed and regulations established vis-à-vis conduct of hikes. The decisions were sent by Dr. Berachiahu to Dr. Eliezer Rieger, the Education Department's supervisor of schools, with a demand that he take it upon himself to ensure their enforcement:

All pupils going out on hikes longer than one day must be checked in advance by the school physician. The doctor will examine Pupil Health Charts and determine who needs a secondary checkup and under what conditions the pupil may participate. A week before the hike, the doctor will receive hike plans. The plans will include places to be visited, location of overnight stops, how many kilometers will be walked each day and how long the hike will last. The doctor will check that places on the itinerary are not infected with contagious diseases. The doctor will provide orders about hygiene regarding sites for overnight stopovers, buying of food and treatment of food bought along the way, and will give orders regarding proper clothing for the season and the location. The doctor will provide a list of medical material to take on the way. A person knowledgeable in administration of first aid will accompany the hike. It is recommended that girls with their period not participate in hikes. On trips [including] girls, at least one female teacher must participate.[183]

Dermatological Treatment and Follow-up

The first school checkups proved that various dermatological diseases — lice, favus, and particularly ringworm — were very prevalent among schoolchildren in Eretz Israel. Prior to surveying activity of the School Hygiene Department in eliminating dermatological diseases in the schools, a brief description of their nature and means of eradication would be appropriate:

Ringworm (tinea capitis, mycosis)

A contagious skin disease of the scalp caused by a type of fungus that causes hair loss. The fungus infects the scalp and hair and does not damage the roots, which remain healthy. After recovery, new, healthy hair grows back. The common treatment was a medicinal salve containing sulfur — unpleasant for both the patient and healthy members of the class. With the introduction of x-ray devices to Hadassah Hospital in Jerusalem, the option to cure ringworm totally and rapidly became available.[184]

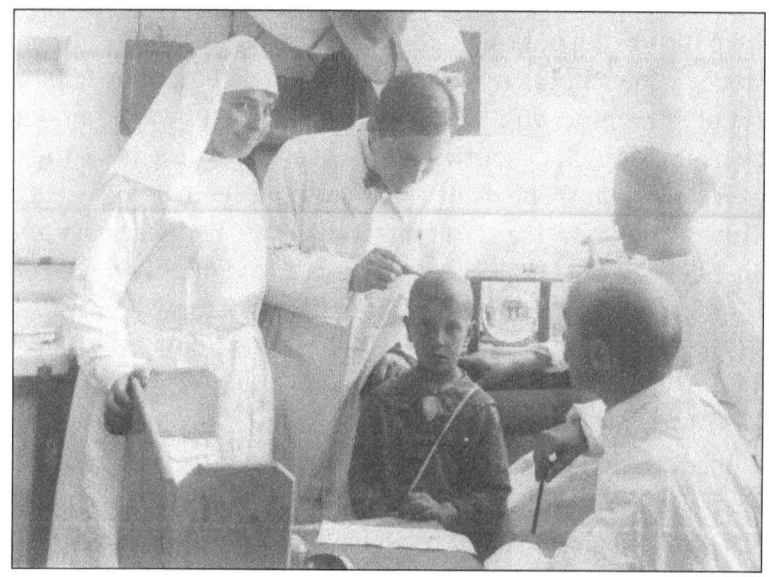

Checking a child head for ringworm, 24% of school children 1920s suffered of ringworm (tinea capitis) (Donchin-Hadassah Collection).

Favus (severe ringworm)

A more severe disease than ringworm in which the fungus destroys the hair roots, leaving the affected area bald for life. The number of children afflicted with favus was much smaller than those afflicted with ringworm. According to examinations carried out by Dr. Arieh Dostrovsky, a school dermatologist, among 4,057 pupils in Jerusalem that he examined in 1926, there were 530 cases of ringworm (13%) and only 52 cases of favus (1.2%).[185]

Lice (pediculosis)

Lice afflicted all schools in frightening proportions and was described as having "become a national affliction in our country."[186] The number of students affected at times encompassed 50–90% of the student body. Other than extensive instruction provided by the School Hygiene Department, practical steps were also taken such as haircuts, special combs and at times suspension from school.

Lack of basic hygienic conditions was conducive to the spread of dermatological diseases. Therefore, under prevailing conditions at the beginning of the twentieth century it was so hard to eradicate them. The School Hygiene Department took upon itself the mission and the struggle to eradicate dermatological diseases and did so methodically and with determined persistence with the assistance of the school physician, the school nurse and the teaching faculty. Curative methods and prophylactic measures taken led to a significant decline in dermatological diseases after only one year of intensive curative work.

Dr. Dostrovsky presented Hadassah management with a detailed report on the prevalence of dermatological disease in schools operated by the Education Committee that reflected the scope of Hadassah's activity in this area and the results achieved. The report encompassed 20 educational institutions in Jerusalem — religious and secular, including kindergartens. All told, 5,733 schoolchildren were examined. Among them, 1,976 were found to be afflicted with ringworm. By the end of the year, 415 (42.5%) had been cured.

By 1928 dermatological diseases were almost totally eradicated from schools operating under the Education Department in Jerusalem, Tel Aviv and Haifa. On the other hand, in other educational institutions such as the religious Talmud Torahs many schoolchildren remained infected with trachoma and ringworm. Dr. Berachiahu warned that regulations set by the School Hygiene Department and followed in other schools — that infected children should be sent home because they serve as a source for spread of the diseases — were not strictly enforced in the Talmud Torah schools. In educational institutions operated by the Education Department, care was taken to isolate infected children, but Dr. Berachiahu noted: "In the Talmud Torahs the administration does not stand on a moral or cultural level and does not take into account the fact that pupils afflicted with ringworm spread the disease among the healthy."[187]

Therefore Dr. Berachiahu called upon the Mandatory government to legislate a law that would encompass all schools and grant school physicians the right to force children with trachoma and ringworm to receive necessary treatment or "to leave the institution until they were cured."[188] Furthermore, while visiting the teachers' seminary in Jaffa, Dr. Berachiahu lectured on dermatological diseases and their treatment and in his closing remarks warned students that if on his next visit to the seminary he found lice, the afflicted students would not be granted teaching certificates.

Ophthalmological Treatment and Follow-up

Hadassah conducted an ongoing and determined struggle with contagious ophthalmological diseases among schoolchildren. The spread of trachoma among pupils reached epidemic proportions. Consequently, the School Hygiene Department introduced systematic eye examinations by an ophthalmologist and daily care for those afflicted with the disease. Those who were cured continued with preventive care within the school framework.

A brief description of trachoma, its nature and steps taken toward its eradication would be appropriate. Trachoma is a contagious disease of the conjunctiva of the eye of viral origin. Signs of the disease are heavy eyelids, a burning sensation and a sense that there is a foreign body irritating the eye, such as a grain of sand, difficulty opening the eye, light tearing and dry pus in the corners of the eye. Those suffering from the disease rub their eyes often and complain of burning and prickling sensations. Untreated, trachoma can cause damage to the cornea that can lead to blindness. Trachoma begins before the patient is aware he has contracted the disease, therefore it constitutes "a disease that is spreading without the patient being aware of his illness."[189] For this reason, it was so important to examine and identify those afflicted with trachoma by methodical examination of all children by an ophthalmologist. Moreover, trachoma is a long-lasting disease that in most forms usually demands systematic, almost monotonous curative care. Therefore doctors often turned treatment over to nurses and paramedics.[190] Methodical curative treatment of trachoma under periodic examination by an experienced doctor brought about a reduction of the number of cases and a restriction of the number of cases with complications.

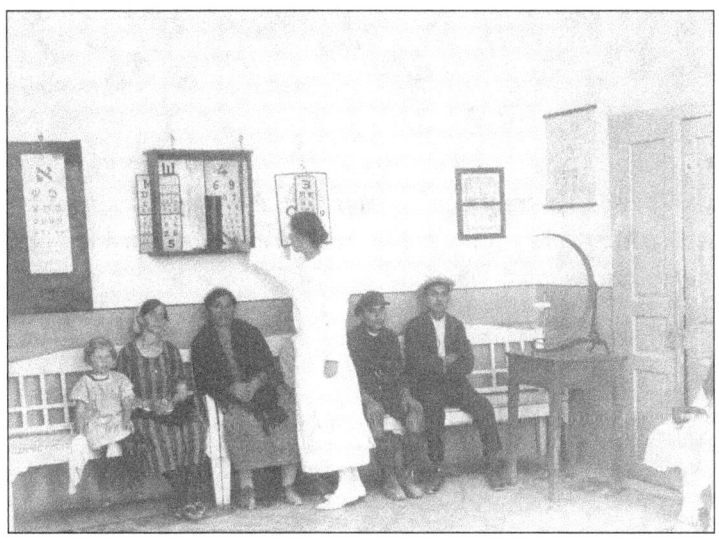

Waiting for an eye checkups in Hadassah clinic (Donchin-Hadassah Collection).

Ophthalmologists argued that trachoma was a difficult disease to eradicate because most patients could not afford to see a doctor due to economic constraints. Dr. Zeev Brunn labeled the disease "the disease of poverty and filth."[191] Dr. Dov-Meir Karinkin clamed "trachoma is for the most part the province of the poor."[192] Likewise, Dr. Chaim Yasski commented that "trachoma is the ailment of the poorest classes and the uncultured."[193]

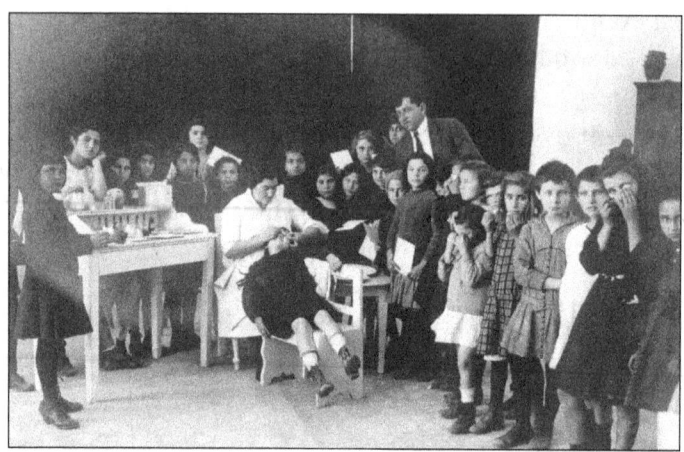

Eye checkups for trachoma, which was the major problem among school children; about 60% of the children in Jerusalem had trachoma (Donchin-Hadassah Collection).

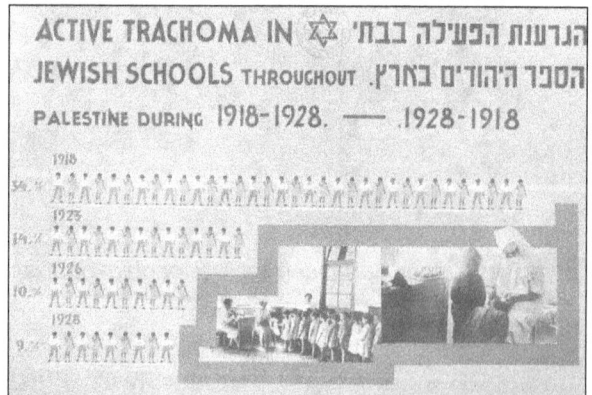

Active Trachoma in Jewish Schools in Eretz Israel 1918-1928 (Donchin-Hadassah Collection).

Trachoma was prevalent among all national and ethic groups in Eretz Israel, but not to the same degree; it was particularly rampant among Arab populations, and less so among locally born Sephardic and Jews. The disease was all the more rare among Ashkenazi immigrants, and almost nonexistent among German-Jewish immigrants. Immigrants from Yemen, on the other hand, suffered in particular from trachoma of all degrees. Due to the contagious nature of the disease, individuals of all ages may contract the disease; however, in Eretz Israel most of those afflicted contracted the disease as young children. Most of those infected were pupils in kindergartens and schools. Therefore, systematic treatment of the disease first began in educational institutions.[194]

The fight against trachoma among schoolchildren was inaugurated in Jerusalem and Tel Aviv prior to the establishment of the School Hygiene Department by Hadassah, but curative care did not encompass all educational institutions in the country, and was not carried out in all cities and agricultural townships (*moshavot*). Three physicians who devoted much time and energy to this effort were Dr. Avraham Ticho, Dr. Arieh Feigenbaum, and Dr. Dov-Meir Karinkin. The three worked in cooperation with the School Hygiene Department.

In accordance with a proposal formulated by Dr. Karinkin, the Hebrew Medical Society in Eretz Israel conducted a survey whose aim was to investigate the scope of the spread of trachoma among Hebrew (i.e., Jewish) educational institutions in the country. Dr. Karinkin presented data and conclusions at the first Trachoma Conference held in 1914 by the Hebrew Medical Society in Eretz Israel. The Conference served as the basis for the formulation of mandatory regulations regarding the disease in educational institutions in the country that stipulated the following: In that trachoma is a long-lasting disease, children should be allowed to attend school, unless their trachoma secretes moisture; those with moist-trachoma would be totally forbidden from attending school; those with dry-trachoma would be allowed to attend school, but must sit on benches in the front of the classroom in order to isolate them as much as possible from the healthy children; those with dry-trachoma would be placed under the supervision of the school physician and curative treatment would be assigned to the school nurse.

Precautionary measures were printed up and posted in classrooms and sent to pupils' homes. In this manner the school did not just cure schoolchildren, but also contributed to the eradication of the disease in the community at large. The posters declared:

Protect Yourself:[195]

1. Wash your hands and face frequently.

2. Avoid bathing in a bathtub used by others.

3. Be very careful not to dry your face with a towel used by others.

4. Avoid touching your eyes with your fingers.

5. Brush flies away from your eyes, nose and mouth.

6. See a doctor immediately if your eyes become red.

In 1920, Dr. Karinkin formulated eye examination guidelines for school physicians regarding trachoma and other contagious ophthalmologic diseases, and sent them to all educational institutions requesting that they be followed:

At the start of the school year, the school doctor would check the eyes of students and teachers. During the year a general examination would be repeated once or twice. Those found infected with moist-trachoma would be temporarily suspended from school until at least partial improvement in their condition, and the trachoma became dry-trachoma.

Children with dry-trachoma would be treated by the school physician. During vacation months treatment would be transferred to a doctor at the General Clinic.

Pupils who were not accepted at school due to moist-trachoma would receive treatment by a doctor at the Pupils' Health Clinic.[196]

Dr. Yehudit Kozlova, an ophthalmologist with the School Hygiene Department, was responsible for curing ophthalmologic diseases among schoolchildren in Jerusalem. Stemming from experience gathered from routine work and general checkups carried out by the schools, she came to two conclusions:

There was a rise in incidence of trachoma at the onset of winter by comparison with the previous spring. This increase influenced the high percentage of patients among new students beginning school in the winter. Thus, trachoma was more prevalent among new students than among the old students who had already received medical care.

At the same time, the number of trachoma cases during the summer months rose among old students due to the effect of summer infections on the spread of trachoma.

Dr. Kozlova came to the conclusion that orderly and methodical curative treatment of infections would reduce the percentage of students infected with trachoma, and prophylactic treatment of infections would serve as preventive care against trachoma by reducing the number of students infected with the disease and would even reduce recurrence of the disease. In Dr. Kozlova's mind, the surest and most radical avenue for prevention of contagious ophthalmologic diseases was "enhancement of the material, cultural and hygienic living conditions of the inhabitants, but these will not easily be changed, therefore other prophylactic measures that can be realized within our state of realities must be employed."[197]

To eradicate trachoma in the schools and the homes of the schoolchildren, Dr. Kozlova recommended the establishment of a special clinic for ophthalmologic care during the summer months to ensure year-round treatment would be ongoing and not disrupted, and that the increasing number of summer infections would be addressed. Dr. Berachiahu succeeded in convincing the Education Committee to allow teachers to supervise treatment "for a lamentable sum," although the Teachers' Federation was in principle opposed to the employment of teachers during the summer vacation.[198] In one of the kindergartens for poor children, in order to maintain regular visits they even gave out cakes "which touched the hearts of all the little ones."[199]

One can learn about the work of the summer eye clinics from a report Dr. Kozlova wrote and sent to Hadassah management in June 1929. Dr. Kozlova described her work at the Contagious Ophthalmologic Disease Clinic in the Old City of Jerusalem. Clinics such as this were established, on her recommendation, in Nachalat Zion and the Bucharian neighborhoods in Jerusalem, which were badly infested with trachoma, and provided treatment for schoolchildren and their families. The program's success prompted Dr. Kozlova to recommend opening clinics year-round, stressing:

> *The summer clinics must become permanent year-round institutions. The work in these clinics must be done [in full cooperation] with work in the schools and the [School] Hygiene Department because only by curing whole families can we achieve truly significant results.*[200]

After three years of work in these clinics, Dr. Kozlova presented a report to Dr. Yasski in which she detailed her achievements in and the results of medical work carried out in the schools and Pupils' Health Clinics in Jerusalem. Dr. Kozlova reported that despite the fact that the scope of trachoma among schoolchildren had been reduced significantly, every year another 300 new active cases in need of medical attention were uncovered among new immigrants from the East (mainly Yemen). Therefore she recommended continuation of treatment of trachoma in the same manner as in the past, and treatment in clinics during the summer months. Her conclusion:

> *An additional step should be taken to eradicate trachoma — in accordance with conditions in our country. It should be attacked from a new front — by curing on a local family-neighborhood basis. For this purpose, local clinics were opened that have proven their importance in the war against trachoma during their brief existence.*[201]

Concurrent with treatment given to pupils in summer clinics and in the schools, Dr. Berachiahu took care to send circulars on a regular basis to school principals and kindergarten teachers to be sure they were enforcing precautionary measures. School physicians joined his efforts: In August 1930 Dr. Arieh Feigenbaum, chief ophthalmologist in the Hadassah Medical Federation, published a "Circular Regarding Ways to Behave In Distancing Children Afflicted with Trachoma from Kindergartens."[202] The circular asked kindergarten teachers to immediately distance children with active trachoma from the kindergarten. But this was not enough. Kindergarten teachers were told to make sure that the children who were temporarily suspended would appear regularly to receive treatment at the clinic, if one existed in their settlement; if not, they themselves were expected to provide treatment on kindergarten premises and ensure the infected child left the kindergarten immediately after receipt of treatment. Dr. Feigenbaum stressed: "One should seize every means so that children secreting pus will not come into contact with other children. After the secretion has passed, they can accept the children back into the kindergarten."[203]

In accordance with this, Dr. Yasski sent a directive to the Education Department in which he told the Department to send an immediate circular to all schools and kindergartens in the cities and *moshavot* instructing pupils afflicted with trachoma to come daily to receive treatment during vacation. At the onset of the school year, the doctors and nurses must present the school principal with a list of children who dodged receipt of treatment during the year or did not show up regularly. To ease the situation for farmers, Dr. Yasski announced: "We will give an order to the doctors and nurses in agricultural locations to arrange ophthalmologic treatment in the evenings, after conclusion of work in the fields.[204]

Annually, Hadassah expended approximately 5,400 Eretz Israel pounds in fighting trachoma. The Mandatory Government Health Department declined to participate in budgeting this work, despite repeated requests from Dr. Berachiahu, Dr. Yasski and Dr. Katzenelson. During the first four years of the Department's operation, the magnitude of the trachoma epidemic was halved, and by the end of the 1930s, the rate of trachoma stood at 3.65%, as illustrated in Chart 2.

Hygienic Supervision and Follow-up of the Schoolchildren, Teachers and Janitors

Hygienic-medical supervision included examination of the cleanliness of the schoolchildren and their clothing; haircuts for needy children as one of the avenues to fight lice and ringworm; monitoring of nutrition and distribution of a glass of hot milk to children suffering from malnutrition; instruction in good hygiene habits such as the use of a toothbrush, handkerchief and personal towel.

In December 1921, Dr. Berachiahu sent a report to Henrietta Szold in which he detailed the difficulties that arose in the process of his

Department supervising hygiene. Among other things, Dr. Berachiahu complained about two central problems and asked Szold to personally intervene: the first was cancellation of funding for haircuts for needy children, and the second, cancellation of funding for hot showers for needy children.

In regard to the haircuts Dr. Berachiahu explained:

> *Shearing hair serves as an excellent weapon in the holy war against lice, scourge of the masses that is being fought worldwide and has yet to be overcome. But the management has found that the 4 pounds a month outlay on this cultural task lays heavy on the budget and one bright day hair cutting was cut.*[205]

In regard to the importance of hot showers, he wrote:

> *Checkups in schools have proven to me that a large number of pupils don't wash their bodies except a number of times a year, and sometimes less than that. Other than what these children carry on themselves constantly in terms of contagious matter of all kinds of diseases that collect on their bodies in their crowded apartments, children of this kind are not normal, are constantly plagued by irritations and can't receive an education in school to an adequate degree. I insisted on installation of hot showers once a week for needy pupils. The joy among the children was tremendous, the air in the classrooms became cleaner and the main thing — I was able to implant a cultured habit of first order: bathing once a week with warm water.*[206]

Dr. Berachiahu asked Szold to take care of allocation of funds for haircuts and showers for children from needy homes to allow for the continuation of this important mission because otherwise "our Department will regress to a very low level."[207] Szold replied in the affirmative and approached the director of Hadassah Medical Federation, Dr. Rubinow, about the matter. In May 1922 she received a reply that a budget of 6 Eretz Israel pounds had been approved for haircuts of children whose parents were not in a financial position to pay.

In the same vein, Dr. Berachiahu turned to the Sanitation Committee of the Tel Aviv Municipality requesting they support his proposal that the city build public showers for schoolchildren. Based on a report by Dr. Borodetzky, a school physician in Tel Aviv, Dr. Berachiahu detailed the necessity and urgency of such a project. The school checkups proved that a large number of pupils took showers very infrequently and the children were filthy. He said:

> ...*The filth contaminates breathing air in the classrooms, filled with children to the gills. An unclean body is accommodating grounds for development of contagious diseases in general, and impedes success in curing eye and skin diseases carried out daily by school nurses. Clean skin is, therefore, a vehicle of first order for the health of the Nation. And the best and cheapest means to a clean body is a shower; therefore we find public showers in all cultured countries as an important reform in raising general hygiene levels of the individual.*[208]

In December 1926, Dr. Berachiahu sent the Education Department a report on hygienic conditions in the schools in which he stressed the importance of adopting a personal towel for each pupil. He cited that in educational institutions where certified nurses worked, there was excellent supervision of this matter, and hygiene measures were strictly maintained. In other schools concern for this matter was in the hands of Health Fellowships. Demands to wash hands and dry them by hygienic use of a personal towel were part of health education that his Department sought to instill in educational institutions. Concurrently, Dr. Berachiahu demanded that school nurses enforce the following hygienic steps:

Ensure each child has a personal towel and handkerchief; send children with colds home for a few days; send children with coughs to be checked by the school physician; teach children in classes not to cough or sneeze, except into a handkerchief; to refrain from visiting public places not under the supervision of teachers and nurses; to take care not to utilize used books and eating utensils; to be sure to wash one's hands before every meal; and not to visit sick schoolmates in their homes.[209]

In his visits to schools, Dr. Berachiahu was in the habit of pointing out defects and hygienic hazards and informing those in charge in order to rectify them. He did not flinch from approaching Hadassah when he encountered refusal to carry out his orders. Thus when Dr. Berachiahu visited the Girls' School in the Old City in Jerusalem and encountered defects that the principal refused to attend to, he sent a wrathful letter to the Eretz Israel Council of Hadassah Women's Federation of America in which he complained that the Girls' School in the Old City prevented providing a supply of water for washing hands before meals; if the school administration continued to stand by their refusal, he would close the cafeteria, he warned.

Dr. Berachiahu demanded and received approval from the Education Department to perform checkups of staff — teachers, kindergarten teachers and janitors — working in schools operated under the auspices of the Education Committee, and a good number of independent Talmud Torah schools. He argued that teachers and janitors were liable to be a source of the spread of contagious diseases among schoolchildren, and therefore they must undergo general checkups by his Department's physicians. As a result of the school physicians' checkups, Dr. Berachiahu issued uniform norms that stipulated: "Teachers whose homes have been afflicted by contagious diseases will not be allowed to enter the school without special permission from the Department."[210] Prior to their acceptance for work in the school, teachers must undergo a thorough medical checkup that includes "tests of urine and feces, to know if the candidate does not carry parasites."[211]

Dr. Berachiahu was stringent about performance of checkups of teaching staff and did not hesitate to release teachers from their posts when it was discovered that they carried diseases. Such was the case when a teacher he checked was found to be suffering from "blood deficiency" (i.e., anemia). Dr. Berachiahu turned to Dr. Yosef Luria, head of the Education Committee, demanding that the teacher be granted a month's sick leave, stipulating:

> ...But on condition that during this time he will receive treatment necessary and will refrain from tasks that put strain on the body. After a month, the teacher should be required to undergo another blood test. When he will be well and return to work, he will be able to teach in the Old City without any damage to his health.[212]

To ensure that all teachers would undergo medical testing, Dr. Berachiahu sent a list of his Department's physicians charged with carrying out checkups to the Education Department, requesting that all teachers, kindergarten teachers and janitors working in Education Department educational institutions be instructed to fulfill this duty: teachers in Jerusalem and its environs by Dr. Berachiahu; teachers in Tel Aviv and its environs by Dr. Borodetzky; teachers in Haifa and its environs by Dr. Rosenberg, teachers in Tiberias and its environs by Dr. Ziss; teachers in Safed and its environs by Dr. Vail.

Hygienic-Sanitary Treatment and Follow-up of Educational Institutions

Most of the buildings where schools and kindergartens for schoolchildren were housed were rented structures. Most were not suitable for their role and furnishing was sparse, old and at times unsuitable. Hygienic-sanitary supervision by the School Hygiene Department included periodic inspections of water supply and quality; cleanliness of classrooms and equipment; the state of furnishings, lighting and ventilation of classrooms; the school yard and fencing; and lavatories, washrooms and plumbing.

School physicians were responsible for sanitary inspections of schools in which they worked. They were accountable for filling out sanitation reports, which were then submitted to Dr. Berachiahu; the director took pains to transfer these reports to the Education Department for rectification of shortcomings.

In a sanitary inspection Dr. Berachiahu carried out in February 1924 at the Tachkemoni School in Jaffa, he found that the school did not meet sanitary standards set by his Department. Dr. Berachiahu listed a host of shortcomings and sent them to the Education Department, stressing: "At the time the new building was rented, I requested that I be consulted in advance in order to rectify shortcomings in time, and to determine the number of pupils in each department (i.e., classroom) in advance."[213]

In a similar sanitary inspection carried in the summer of 1926 by Tel Aviv school physician Dr. Borodetzky in the Talpiot School — an ultra-orthodox *haredi* girls' school in Tel Aviv — many shortcomings were found. These included lack of gymnastics, a lunchroom, showers — or at least a washroom, sufficient stalls in the toilets for 400 pupils and other deficiencies.[214]

Due to the importance of the issue, Dr. Berachiahu addressed hygiene and sanitation planning of school premises on the agenda of the national convention of school physicians that took place in Jerusalem on April 1, 1928. He approached architect Fritz Kornburg, requesting that he lecture on the subject of "the modern school building in Eretz Israel from the viewpoint of the architect."[215]

Dr. Berachiahu did not satisfy himself with merely arranging the lecture, but also sent a letter to the Society of Engineers and Architects in Eretz Israel inviting them to the convention, citing: "The lecture and ensuing deliberations must clarify theoretical questions whose solution is very important for the development of schools. Subsequently, it would be most desirable if the honorable engineers and architects would participate in this convention."[216]

Indeed, two weeks before the opening of the conference, a reply was received from Chairman A. Kook, president of the Society of Engineers and Architects in Eretz Israel, in which he informed Dr. Berachiahu of their participation in the convention.

Decisions made at this conference included issues tied to school structures. The following decision was made: "School buildings: The Education Department shall arrange a permanent committee for approval of plans for school buildings and their building lots. Construction of a school building will not be begun without approval of all details by the above committee."[217]

On the authority of the decision, Dr. Berachiahu turned to the Education Department warning them "not to make any concessions"[218] in the planning of schools, as was done at the time of the building of toilets in the Tachkemoni and Lamel schools. Over this matter an acrimonious debate broke out between Dr. Berachiahu and the architects. Dr. Berachiahu demanded that toilets face the sun "and for this reason should not be constructed on two sides with a corridor down the middle, because in this arrangement only one side can get enough sun." Dr. Berachiahu based his demand on a publication of the United States Public Health Service where it was written that "toilet rooms should be well ventilated and should be so situated that the sunlight will enter them during part of the day."

Dr. Berachiahu argued:

> *If in America this is so, in a spot where there is not only water for rinsing and soap for cleaning, but where toilets are cleaned with hot water, while here on one hand we don't have such means and on the other hand we are plagued by flies, which are far from easy to fight, and there are among our children many who suffer from parasites expelled in human excrement, our previous demand vis-à-vis toilet facilities is all the more important to fulfill.*[219]

In closing, Dr. Berachiahu concluded: "There should be no capitulation to concessions as we did in the above two institutions under pressure from the architects. As for aesthetic questions, I don't discount them at all, let the architects discuss and make efforts to find a suitable solution, but not one at the expense of hygiene."[220]

Indeed in January 1930, the Education Department approached Dr. Berachiahu requesting his evaluation of plans for new buildings. Dr. Berachiahu responded immediately, saying "this is the duty of my post."[221] Dr. Berachiahu seized the moment to warn that the Education Department had again rented new buildings for schools without consulting his Department first, as had been done in the Girl's Seminary and Girls' School.

He reprimanded the principal of the Girls' School, saying: "I am surprised that you moved to a new building and did not think it necessary to invite me, neither before nor after the move, to consult on necessary alterations. At present I don't know if the room you allocated as a lunchroom is truly suitable or not."[222]

The state of school buildings was bad not only in Jerusalem and Tel Aviv, but also in smaller settlements. This fact is reflected in a sanitary survey conducted by Dr. Mirenburg, a traveling ophthalmologist who covered schools in settlements all over the Galilee and the environs of Haifa — Rosh Pina and Chittin in the Upper Galilee, Achziv in the Western Galilee, Nahalal in the Jezreel Valley to Nesher and Atlit, respectively east and south of Haifa. From her survey one can appreciate the stark sanitary conditions of schools on the periphery where neglect, shabbiness and distress prevailed; in Rosh Pina the first grade was housed in a structure that had previously served as a dairy barn and was altered to serve as a classroom. The structure "lacked a floor and was surrounded by manure and flies." In the other settlement school children studied under very crowded conditions in tiny rooms that barely held their occupants. The doctor's primary complaint was the state of sanitation in toilets. In Chittin, "the sanitary situation is terrible. Toilets are in a state of cleanliness inferior by any standard." In Atlit, "the sanitary condition of toilets is very bad. Plumbing is broken. Water is stagnant and this can cause all kinds of diseases."[223]

The harsh state of hygiene in educational facilities was raised again and again in discussions and meetings of school nurses. In a meeting of nurses in Jerusalem, the nurses complained that it was difficult to make children wash their hands after using the toilet and before eating because the schools lacked provisions for doing so. Dr. Berachiahu promised to approach the Education Department "about arranging sinks in the schools near the toilets, and placing newspaper in the toilets and pails for paper."[224]

A month later, the subject was raised again among Jerusalem nurses. It was decided:

Because it is indispensable that in lower grades washing hands be conducted in the classroom and not at the yard washbasin, a sink should be arranged in the classroom.

The nurses should be responsible for arranging little bags from cloth that are divided in two: one side for a towel to dry hands before eating, the other side for another towel, to dry hands after using the toilet."[225]

At the same meeting it was also decided to request the Education Department "to arrange pergolas in schools that don't have shaded areas to allow ventilation of the classrooms and the meeting hall, and so the pupils will not spend every recess under a hot summer sun."[226]

Supervision of Janitors

The work of the janitors occupied an important role in the general work of the School Hygiene Department. Therefore Dr. Berachiahu placed great importance on professional organization of janitors who worked in educational institutions. He was even in the habit of participating, at their invitation, in the national convention of janitors, and lecturing before them on the importance of maintaining sanitation and hygiene in educational institutions. It became evident that this did not help, for in his many visits to educational institutions throughout the country, Dr. Berachiahu was appalled by the lack of hygiene, filth and neglect in schoolyards, in classrooms and particularly in the toilets. His repeated complaints and protests to Dr. Berkson, director of the Education Department, about the slovenly and irresponsible work done by the janitors and their unsuitability to their role fell on deaf ears. Dr. Berkson replied: "A good portion of the shortcomings of the janitors can be rectified only by enhancing their economic state. If a janitor could attain a salary of 9–10 Eretz Israel pounds, we would find more suitable people."[227]

In May 1932, a prolonged strike broke out in educational institutions lasting eleven days. The hygienic-sanitary situation, which was terrible to begin with, became unbearable in many educational institutions. Dr. Berachiahu was forced to warn that the state of sanitation constituted a health hazard to pupils and teachers, and if the toilets were not cleaned immediately, schools would have to be closed forthwith. He informed Dr. Berkson that "continuation of studies under present conditions was certain to inflict damage to the health of children."[228] Dr. Berachiahu cited that only in schools where Health Fellowships carried out regular work were conditions reasonable, for the Fellowships took care of cleaning the classrooms, but on the other hand they were labeled "strike breakers" by the janitors, "a horrible label in the eyes of educators and their wards."[229]

In a January 1932 meeting of the Committee for Investigation of Operative Avenues of the School Hygiene Department, Dr. Berachiahu raised the problem of the poor performance of the janitors, putting his complaints on the table:

...Their work is very bad...the janitors in the Mizrachi institutions
are all unsuitable...We suggested several years ago not to accept janitors
without the agreement of the principal of the institution and the Hygiene
Department, and each janitor must undergo an apprenticeship under an
experienced janitor...Janitors don't know janitorship. They come to school
late and hire irresponsible substitutes....[230]

The janitor problem was raised in numerous meetings of school physicians and nurses and complaints were brought before directors of Education Departments in various cities throughout the country, in the hopes that they, with the authority they wielded, would be able to assist. In Tel Aviv the nurses initiated a meeting with Dr. Yitzhak Alterman, director of the Education Department, and complained about the poor performance of the janitors. After hearing their claims, Dr. Alterman suggested that each nurse put her complaints in writing, have the principal sign the complaint and refer it to him. Dr. Alterman promised to discuss all the complaints with the director of the Education Department in Jerusalem. The situation deteriorated when one of the principals refused to sign the complaint and even told the janitor about it. The janitor replied in a letter to the director labeling the nurse a "murderer." The school physician was forced to defend the nurse, and wrote to Dr. Berachiahu: "If to fight dirt in the schools the Hygiene Department must deal not only with the janitors but also with the principals, it's no surprise that results of the war in a number of schools are zero."[231]

Dealing with the "janitor problem" continued to occupy Dr. Berachiahu for many years, until the passage of the Janitors' Work Law by the Education Department. School principals and school medical staff accepted the legislation and demanded it be enforced. A good number of problems were solved with the establishment of new, modern and better-equipped schools.

Despite objective and subjective stumbling blocks — from lack of funding to lack of experience, absence of collaboration due to power struggles and personality clashes, and the normal and expectable tensions common to any institution in the "process of becoming" in historical prospective — we are witnesses to the formulation and realization, for the first time, of an organized system for providing medical services to schoolchildren and teaching staff in Eretz Israel — a system organized and occupied by professionals that established health and hygiene standards for schoolchildren and their families. For the first time in their lives, pupils received systematic medical services within the confines of their schools, while strictly maintaining daily treatment orders to overcome contagious diseases that were prevalent in Eretz Israel at the time.

D. Mental Hygiene Work

School hygiene was designed not only to prevent diseases that could be detrimental to the development of the child, but also to uncover positive and negative factors in the psychological maturation progress of the child in his studies and social adjustment. Thus, among the roles adopted by the School Hygiene Department was clarification of the roots of social maladjustment, as a factor in personality disorders and mental illness.

Mental hygiene as a field was not sufficiently developed in the 1920s. Only with the arrival of a wave of Jewish physicians from Germany in the 1930s in the wake of Hitler's rise to power, did mental hygiene begin to witness rapid development. At the end of 1935, these doctors from Germany constituted half of the medical community in Eretz Israel; it was a peak immigration year that led to a surplus of doctors in the country.[232] One of the outstanding characteristics of this wave of immigration was the expertise of its physicians. At the time of their arrival, medicine in Eretz Israel was based on general medicine. In general, hospitalization services were on an elementary level and characterized by a low level of specialization. The doctors from Germany, most of them experts in their chosen fields, changed the face of medicine in the country.[233]

Among the experts who emigrated from Germany were psychiatrists who established psychiatric departments within the framework of general hospitals and Kupat Holim's central clinics. The mental health field was particularly advanced among Jewish doctors in Germany and Austria, and one of the most backward fields of medicine in Eretz Israel at the time.

Up until 1933, there was only one psychiatric hospital in the country — *Ezrat Nashim*[234] (Women's Aid) in Jerusalem, directed by Dr. Heintz Hermann.[235] Routine treatment of the mentally ill was usually limited to hospitalization in closed institutions, designed to protect society from the inmates. In 1933, the psychiatrists from Germany joined Dr. Hermann, and in 1934 they established a professional organization together — the Society of Neuropsychiatry —that embraced all those engaged in mental health work in Eretz Israel.[236]

Care of "problematic and exceptional" or mentally disabled children had yet to be established. The first institutions designed for this purpose were designated for both trainable and unattainable, together in one place.[237] They were established by the church or charitable persons prompted by humanitarian motivations and genuine concern for the welfare of the children. The primary goal of these philanthropic endeavors was to assist the parents and free them as much as possible from the burden of caring for the children and solve the problem of their education.

In view that there were not yet suitable frameworks for such children, the School Hygiene Department headed by Dr. Berachiahu took upon itself the mission of caring for these children as an integral part of the Department's educational-health work. Dr. Berachiahu differentiated between two categories among the children: hard-to-educate children and retarded children. He defined the two groups thus: "A retarded child is one who is mentally impaired; a hard-to-educate child is a child with a defect in his personality, in his behavior."[238]

In his opinion, the most suitable care for retarded children was to integrate them into a special school whose purpose was to provide for the child's basic needs. Suitable care for hard-to-educate children was to integrate them into boarding school frameworks — such as the youth villages operating at Ben Shemen and Shfeyah[239] — where they could live and study together with other children their age.

Dr. Berachiahu's adoption of this kind of solution was based on two theories: The first was held by German immigrant psychiatrists who claimed that "in Berlin they have ceased sending hard-to-educate children to foster families for care, and preferred to send them to children's institutions."[240] The second was the widely held theory that environment, along with genetic factors, was a decisive factor in the normal development of the child. The child was not only influenced by his surroundings, but was built by them. He was exposed — almost without the ability to resist, and particularly at a tender age — to the persuasive and formative power of his surroundings. A Spartan, crowded and poverty-stricken environment open to disease and neglect was liable to produce phenomena of retardation, lead to mental disturbance and stunt normal growth and development. By removing the child from this environment and placing him in a progressive and supportive educational environment, it was possible to help him overcome future difficulties.[241]

At the beginning, the School Hygiene Department dealt with exceptional children on an individual basis. Such children were identified by teachers, parents, school nurses and school physicians and referred for counseling, testing, guidance and treatment by the Hygiene Department. With the rise in the number of exceptional children (hard-to-educate, mentally retarded, abandoned and delinquent children) in the school system, two needs became apparent: on one hand, the need to find a suitable frameworks outside the regular school; on the other hand, the need to address the mental hygiene of all schoolchildren in the school system in a professional manner.

Care of Hard-to-Educate Children

A significant change in the care of exceptional children began in 1929 with the opening of a Consultation Station (termed a "heal-pedagogical" station)[242] by the School Hygiene Department. This was the first of its kind in the country to care for hard-to-educate children and children with adjustment problems, or as Dr. Berachiahu expressed it:

> This was the first and only of its kind, not only in Eretz Israel, but also in surrounding countries. And children and youth were sent to it for testing and treatment, not only from various corners of our country, but also from neighboring countries: from Syria and Egypt.[243]

In order to open the Consultation Station in Jerusalem, the Department was in need of additional budgeting. Dr. Berachiahu turned to Hadassah in America requesting additional funding, but much to his surprise, at the same time Dr. Bluestone, director of Hadassah in Eretz Israel, approached him to offer financing. Dr. Berachiahu praised the unexpected initiative, saying:

> *I can never forget this merciful act of Hadassah management on behalf of [furthering] development of the School Hygiene Department's work, when it accepted my proposal to establish a station to treat hard-to-educate children.*[244]

The beginnings were unassuming, but significant: The Consultation Station was established in the Straus Health House in Jerusalem, to treat children "with normal intelligence abilities, but defective from an emotional aspect."[245] Children with various disturbances such as stuttering, anxieties, aggressiveness, stealing, lack of appetite, tics, insomnia, learning difficulties, neuroses and so forth, were referred. Parents from outside Jerusalem also turned to the Station for assistance.

Work at the Consultation Station was arranged as follows:

Preliminary diagnosis was the prerogative of kindergarten teachers and schoolteachers, based on observation of the child, relying on the educator's knowledge and pedagogic experience to identify schoolchildren who appeared "suspect" of any kind of anomaly.

Referral of the pupil to the school physician, through the auspices of the school nurse.

Examination of the pupil by the school physician. After confirmation of the educators' diagnosis, referral to the Consultation Station. The physician filled in a questionnaire to receive updated information on the pupil, his personal data and description of the anomaly. The questionnaire was filled out with care under Dr. Berachiahu's guidance: "One should refrain from short utterances that are meaningless, such as: The child is a thief, lazy, hot-tempered, and so forth, in lieu of supplying examples of these things."[246] The questionnaire was kept in a special file together with medial checkups and psychological tests, and all other documentation including grades, essays and so forth done by the child.

Physical checkup and intelligence testing of the child by a medical specialist at the Consultation Station, and formulation of a diagnosis and recommended treatment.

Treatment, twice a week per pupil in the afternoon hours. From time to time, parents and pupil were invited for discussion, guidance and consultation regarding arrangement for placement in an institution or integration of the child in occupational work of some kind.

Due to a shortage of teaching staff trained in special education, Dr. Berachiahu sent three schoolteachers for special training in heal-pedagogical in Vienna, under the auspices of Hadassah and financed by WIZO (Women's International Zionist Organization) in Vienna. One of the three was subsequently asked to manage the Consultation Station in Jerusalem. Within a short time, hard-to-educate schoolchildren were being referred to the Station from throughout the country. The need for another Station became evident. Indeed, two years later, in 1931, a second Consultation Station was opened in Tel Aviv, thus providing similar services to inhabitants of the *moshavot* south of Tel Aviv and in the Sharon region, to bring their children for testing, counseling and guidance. Schoolteachers also turned to the Consultation Stations to receive counseling on how to deal with children with behavioral problems.

Over time, Dr. Berachiahu sought to integrate mental hygiene work more professionally within the framework of the School Hygiene Department by appointing a doctor who was a specialist in mental illness as director of mental hygiene and by soliciting special funding to develop this medical branch. To achieve this, he initiated a meeting with Dr. Yasski, Hadassah's director, and Dr. Elchanan Rabinowitz,[247] a pediatrician, to formulate a work program and ways to put it into practice.

At the meeting, Dr. Berachiahu described his Department's work in mental hygiene that he had begun nine years earlier in 1921, suggesting that the time was ripe to expand this important work — by assigning it to a physician trained in the field and formalizing mental hygiene work as an integral part of the work of the School Hygiene Department. Dr. Yasski agreed that "this new branch of our work is tightly tied to the work of the School Hygiene Department."[248] He requested that Dr. Rabinowitz serve as head, under the direct supervision of Dr. Berachiahu.

Dr. Rabinowitz agreed to take the task upon himself, but only after presenting his own personal credo: "Mental hygiene is the study of the child's psyche. One must know his individual well and to do so, one must penetrate the school and the home."[249]

When Dr. Rabinowitz learned that he would be expected to engage in mental hygiene alongside routine medical work in the schools, he asked that he be relieved of the duties of school physician claiming that he was not well enough acquainted with general hygiene work, and that implementation of the detailed plan he had prepared would not leave enough time to deal with ongoing hygiene problems. The meeting closed with the decision that medical responsibility for two Jerusalem schools — Tachkemoni and Lamel — would be turned over to Dr. Rabinowitz, but stipulated:

> ...Under the condition that he would carry out all the duties of the school physician required by the Hygiene Department that included: examination of heads for signs of ringworm [and] lice, while taking note of hygiene of apparel, sleep and nutrition, that should be given attention, for in the end analysis, they were the foundations for mental hygiene.[250]

Being subordinate to Hadassah management and the Education Department, Dr. Berachiahu was in the habit of regularly sending his superiors detailed reports, memorandums and updates about the ongoing work of his Department that allowed the recipients to stay abreast of developments in the School Hygiene Department, its achievements and difficulties encountered. For Dr. Berachiahu, the reports served three purposes: To inform his superiors of all aspects of the Department's work; to attempt to involve others in the difficulties encountered in application of his program, in order to request assistance in the form of additional personnel and funding; and to attempt to increase the Department's budget.

From the reports, the development of mental hygiene work in Eretz Israel, and the urgent need for this work, became evident. Consultation Stations were established in Jerusalem, Tel Aviv and Haifa in the north. The stations were operated in part with Hadassah funding and in part with funding provided by the residents.

The "Emek" Consultation Station established in the north in the Jezreel Valley provided services to schoolchildren in the *kibbutzim* and *moshavot* Kfar Yechezkel, Ein Harod, Tel Yosef and Beit Alfa and was funded by the communities themselves. In Tel Aviv and Haifa, Stations were also operated by residents, serving nearby settlements as well. The Stations were located on school premises, as was customary in the United States. The work of the Stations with "criminal children, those who wet their beds at night, stuttered, children who refused to eat and so forth among hard-to-educate children"[251] proved fruitful, but constituted a budgetary burden on the School Hygiene Department. Consequently, Dr. Berachiahu requested a budget of 12 Eretz Israel pounds per month for the Jerusalem Station; only 6 pounds were requested for the Tel Aviv Station, because in Tel Aviv, parents participated in covering the operating costs. Dr. Berachiahu hoped that his request would be honored, for he stressed that he had invested "so much effort and energy and had reached a high level of development."[252] Jerusalem required a particularly good Station, because students at the seminars — future teachers — visited the Station to gain practical experience through observation.

Letters and protocols found among archival material shed light on the kinds of educational solutions found for those schoolchildren referred to the Consultation Stations. It becomes evident that the primary goals of the School Hygiene Department in its mental hygiene work were to diagnose mentally disabled children as early as possible, preferably in kindergarten, and to plan a suitable rehabilitative-educational program for the child that would allow him, when the time came, to be successfully employed, without becoming a burden on his family or the public purse — that is, to prepare him for a productive life as a member of modern society.

At the beginning of the 1930s, Hadassah policy underwent a change. In the wake of deteriorating finances within the organization stemming from the Great Depression in the United States, the organization began to transfer most of its medical facilities outside Jerusalem to Kupat Holim or municipal auspices. Policy changes were also registered in the School Hygiene Department.

On July 1, 1930, Hadassah management suggested that within the framework of "plans for cuts in [the] School Hygiene Department's 1932 budget," the Jerusalem Heal-Pedagogical Station in Jerusalem be closed. Dr. Berachiahu was adamantly opposed to such a move, claiming:

> *There is no similar work being done in Eretz Israel. With great efforts, I succeeded in establishing a Station in Jerusalem, and it can be a praise to Hadassah work in general, of which we have the perfect right to be proud.*[253]

Dr. Berachiahu succeeded in staving off the dreaded decree, and the Jerusalem Station continued to operate. More than that, by 1946 two more Consultation Stations had been established in Jerusalem, and with the assistance of the Tel Aviv Municipality, a school for special education had been established in Tel Aviv.

Care of Retarded Children

The question of care of retarded children bothered Dr. Berachiahu greatly, and he aspired to establish a special institution for them, based on his belief that their rehabilitation was possible only in a special school and only upon receipt of suitable educational care that was geared to their needs. Because the financial resources of the School Hygiene Department were limited, while needs were great, Dr. Berachiahu knew that without mobilization of special funding and massive financial assistance, he could not realize his plans. For this purpose, he approached the Education Department and the Education Committee suggesting that mental hygiene work be integrated as part of the general work of the Education Department, and proposed the establishment of institutions for the retarded, throughout the country. When his requests solicited no response, Dr. Berachiahu complained to Hadassah management that it would be possible to achieve more with retarded children:

> *...If the Education Department would also take upon itself the duty of treating this serious and painful problem, or at least would assist the Hygiene Department, it would not be left alone in the battle in its search and its endeavors.*[254]

When he came to the conclusion that the Education Department would not assist in establishing a school for the retarded, he turned to people of influence in the Yishuv in order to obtain funding to establish and operate such an institution.

At first, Dr. Berachiahu approached Dr. Reuven Katzenelson, deputy director general of Hadassah. He responded that he had received Dr. Berachiahu's interesting memorandum regarding the urgent need to open an institution for educating retarded children, adding that he had referred his proposal to Hadassah in the United States and when a response was received, he would pass it on to Dr. Berachiahu. Aware that such a process could take time, Dr. Berachiahu turned to Shoshana Persitz, head of the Education Department of the Tel Aviv Municipality. His appeal generated interest. Persitz approached a number of affluent families with retarded children, and with the assistance of the Municipality, in 1929 a school for educable and trainable — the first of its kind in Eretz Israel — was organized.

The institution was under the supervision of the Education Department of the National Committee (*Va'ad Haleumi*) and the School Hygiene Department. Its beginnings were modest — only two classes with two teachers, an assistant, a cook and a nursemaid. The teachers had undergone professional training — one in Vienna, the other in Russia. The assistant was a graduate of the Tel Aviv Teachers' Seminary. Dr. Berachiahu picked the students. A pedagogic committee was organized to serve the school, and comprised Mina Grumann, school principal; Dr. Yitzhak Alterman, supervisor of kindergartens in Eretz Israel; Dr. Yosef Ozerkovsky-Azaryahu, supervisor of schools in the Judea Region; and Dr. Berachiahu.

At the outset, "The School for Retarded Children" began with only 12 children. The School was so small that it could accept only a small number of those in need from among all those who sought to apply. Mina Grumann — one of the three women sent to Vienna to study special education — was appointed principal. Within a year, the student body was increased to 24 students, and within two years reached 42 children, divided into four classes in a five-room building. In order to expand the teaching faculty, two more teachers were sent to Berlin to study special education among retarded children. Upon their return to Eretz Israel one in 1931, the other in 1933 — the two began teaching.

Teaching methods adopted by the School for Retarded Children were based on a preference for instilling concrete knowledge before theoretical knowledge. Therefore, studies were tailored to individual needs and dictated by the living environment of each pupil in the program. The teaching principles adopted were based on the child's disabilities. Among the fundamental guiding principles embraced:

- Concrete illustration of material learned.

- A focused study approach to subject matter.

- Concentration on subjects taken from the child's immediate surroundings.

The goal was to instill the children with life habits within a healthy society, equip them with occupational skills, and distance them from neglect and crime. This was the initial goal, but it quickly became evident that many children in need of this educational framework could not be integrated for lack of space. To reduce the burden, in the meantime, special classes were opened within regular existing schools — based on a special curriculum for exceptional children, in which handicrafts occupied a central role.

In 1935, Principal Mina Grumann sent a memorandum to the Tel Aviv Municipality's Education and Culture Department regarding the School for Retarded Children. In the memorandum she surveyed the history of the institution from its beginnings, and the difficulties that accompanied the School's operation and impeded development and expansion. Grumann cited that 100 applications had been submitted that year, but only 30 could be accepted due to lack of space. The number of students accepted was merely a small proportion of the retarded children living in Tel Aviv. Moreover, the School lacked workshops for subjects such as carpentry, sewing and shoe repair and did not have an orderly kitchen or a small agricultural farm,[255] and thus the School could not help the children learn any trade.[256]

In addition, the facility suffered from lack of a suitable building and had inadequate furnishing. The principal requested to expand the School to allow acceptance of more children. Her proposal called for adding three classes and increasing the size of the faculty. All of Grumann's plans, however, were rejected due to lack of funding. The principal had closed her memorandum in a tone of reproach, stating: "An institution existing some six years that has proved its ability is surely worthy that a school [building] should be established for it. Therefore it is most particular that all plans in this matter have gone nowhere."[257]

A year later, Grumann wrote a second memorandum to the Tel Aviv Municipality, from which one may learn that most of her plans were not carried out. The number of schoolchildren in her facility still stood at 40 and the school staff had not grown at all. This memorandum also closed with words of reproach:

> It is high time that the first school [for retarded children] in the country will be rectified, that it should be finished and improved according to its function. It's time that those responsible for education of the younger generation will recognize that any further neglect or any delay, will come back to take revenge upon us.[258]

Nevertheless, there was some progress elsewhere. In 1934 a second School for Retarded Children was opened in Petach Tikva, east of Tel Aviv, but its fate was no better than that of the first.

Care of Abandoned and Delinquent Children

In 1931, the Delegate Assembly of the National Assembly (Asefat Hanivcharim shel Knesset Israel) — the representative body of the Yishuv — established a network of social welfare services in Eretz Israel that encompassed social work. Henrietta Szold stood at the head of the Social Work Department that operated within the framework of the National Committee. In this capacity, Szold was also responsible for Jewish juvenile delinquents. In the process of dealing with these children, Szold discovered that most of the children under her Department's care were abandoned children — only some of them were delinquents. Szold turned to Dr. Berachiahu, expressing her hopes that their departments could collaborate in dealing with these children.

The School Hygiene Department agreed to take it upon itself to deal with delinquent youth, together with the National Committee's Social Work Department. Dr. Berachiahu was even appointed a member of a committee that dealt with the problem of their rehabilitation; the committee was established in 1932 by the National Committee, and first convened on June 14, 1932, in Jerusalem. The body was composed of the following individuals: Yosef Meyuchas, an educator and supervisor of playgrounds in Jerusalem; Rachel Schwartz, a supervisor of playgrounds in Eretz Israel; Jurist K. Friedenburg; A. Avizohar; Beba Idelson; A. Yafe; and Szold. Jurist Rosa Ginsburg was appointed chairperson of the committee. Szold, head of the National Committee's Social Work Department, opened the meeting with a survey of the intensive work invested by her Department, together with the School Hygiene Department, in rehabilitation of juvenile delinquents to date.

The contents of her survey revealed that work in Tel Aviv and Jerusalem gradually expanded as a result of the large number of children-at-risk. She cited in particular that "...criminal children whose number have grown and grown of late, and that the courts have sentenced them to banishment to a school for [juvenile] felons, a place from which they are sure to come out anti-social human beings."[259]

Szold came to an agreement with Mr. Reynolds, government administrator for juvenile delinquents, that the Mandatory official would not request their incarceration in reform schools, under the condition that the youths would receive supervision and treatment. Therefore, Szold had these children transferred to the authority of the School Hygiene Department for treatment, with the assumption that the Department would attend to their rehabilitation. There were, however, youths who despite these efforts had to be sent to the school for juvenile offenders in Tul Karem, an Arab village northeast of Tel Aviv. This reform school, established in 1923, was a government-run reformatory designed for both Jewish and Arab offenders.[260] The institution was in the habit of imposing harsh punishments — a state of affairs that prompted the Jerusalem branch of the Teachers' Federation to intervene, and even to call upon the National Committee "to take steps to abolish whipping as a punishment for these children."[261] Szold met with Reynolds in order to learn about the reformatory, its arrangements, the number of students and the educational approach it employed.

According to Szold's findings, the following picture emerged: Examination of the social welfare status of these children revealed that the majority were hard cases with two primary factors that had influenced the children to commit crimes — their harsh economic straits that resulted in their inability to pay tuition and therefore they roamed the streets "and associate[d] with dishonest society,"[262] and their psychological deficiencies.

Szold requested that the committee discuss the problems of these children and suggest effective avenues that should be taken vis-à-vis the legal, educational and social-welfare aspects of the problem at hand. She requested the committee's members to give their expert opinions regarding the method she favored — assigning "Big Brothers"[263] to befriend these children and act as positive role models and mentors.

Dr. Berachiahu expressed his opinion that treatment of delinquent children should be divided into three areas: judicial-legal; medical-pedagogic and social.

In his estimation, there were a number of reasons for delinquency. The first was mistakes in upbringing, deficiencies in family life, social neglect and so forth — this reason applied to the majority of cases. The second was defects in intelligence, but these were the minority. Dr. Berachiahu cited that a portion of crimes, such as theft and sex crimes, were perpetrated in periods of mental crises such as adolescence or early puberty. Treatment of these cases belonged to heal-pedagogical stations. Children of the first category could be rehabilitated through proper treatment at heal-pedagogical stations, but children of the second category could not be reformed except in special schools that endeavored to advance the child through heal-pedagogy. In Dr. Berachiahu's professional opinion, a school that did not try to reform the child in this manner, inflicted damage — both by administration of unsuitable education and by marring the child's future by tagging him a "criminal" wherever he turned. One of the most important tools in reform and treatment was observation stations. Dr. Berachiahu opposed the creation of special institutions for delinquent children because in his estimation, some should be left in the custody of their family. On the other hand, some must be removed from "the family atmosphere" and should be placed with a foster family or a residential educational facility. The most effective means was work arrangements for such youths, particularly in kibbutzim.

Dr. Berachiahu suggested establishment of three committees to address treatment of delinquent children:

The *Judicial-Legal Committee* whose role would be defense of the child in court and prevention of placement in reform school, unless recommended by a team of medical specialists.

The *Medical-Pedagogic Committee* whose role would be to cure the child by suitable treatment — dealing with both the child and his environment (family, parents). Psychiatrists working with the committee in an advisory capacity would provide diagnosis and choice of treatment framework: either the School for Retarded Children in Tel Aviv or the Consultation Station ("heal-pedagogical" station) in Jerusalem or Tel Aviv. The committee was to be composed of a physician trained in heal-pedagogy, a psychiatrist and a member of the Social Welfare Committee.

The *Social Welfare Committee* whose role would be to receive input from the Medical-Pedagogic Committee and seek avenues to carry out its instructions, in one of the following ways: 1) Placement of the retarded child in the school for retarded children. 2) Transfer of the child to a foster family or educational institution. 3) Appointment of a guardian for the child during treatment. 4) Location of a place of work, as an avenue for treatment tool — on a farm, in an office or in a workshop.

Members of the National Committee supported Szold's approach that called for supervision of young delinquents by assigning Big Brothers and Dr. Berachiahu's idea to adopt a work-oriented rehabilitation program on kibbutzim or *moshav* farms, or placement in a suitable agricultural school such as the Ben Shemen and Meir Shfeyah youth villages. Other ideas were also raised such as integration of the children in youth movements or playgrounds.[264]

Public bodies — first and foremost the National Committee — demanded that the British Mandatory government establish a reformatory in a Jewish settlement and authorize the courts to send young Jewish delinquents there, when necessary. The committee argued that the Tul Karem reformatory was suitable for Arab children, but not Jewish children since the language of instruction was Arabic. Moreover, they added: "All the inside arrangements are non-Jewish in a way that makes it impossible to receive national or religious education, or instill habits in accordance with Judaism."[265]

Dr. Berachiahu, who visited the reformatory, said that:

> The food is not kosher and the children know they are eating non-kosher food. From a pedagogic-educational standpoint, this is a great mistake. The children become accustomed to sinning forced upon them from above. This is a kind of direct tutelage in sin and delinquency.[266]

In the second meeting of the Committee for Rehabilitation of Delinquents held two weeks later on June 28, 1932, the suggestions raised in the first meeting were reviewed. Operative methods were formulated and adopted. Committee member A. Friedenburg, a legal attorney, suggested asking the chief of police to provide information on Jewish children at the Tul Karem reformatory. Each case should subsequently be reviewed to ascertain if there were children among them who "could be reformed outside this reform school."[267] Friedenburg also suggested appealing to the most senior judge or the secretary of the court, requesting that they order all judges to take into account that the Tul Karem school "still does not stand on an appropriate level"[268] and they should refrain as much as possible from sending children there, release children on bail and abolish beatings as punishment. At the meeting three committees were chosen; each committed itself to discuss the issue and formulate suggestions. Recommendations were presented to the Committee for Rehabilitation of Delinquents chairperson, attorney Rosa Ginzberg, who in turn submitted a comprehensive memorandum on the issue to Szold. The memorandum was brought before the National Social Welfare Council, discussed and passed on to the National Committee for a final judgment.

The following decisions were made: A reform school for delinquent Jewish youth would be established adjacent to the Kaduri Agricultural

School, so that the children would be in a Hebrew environment, receive Jewish education and study agriculture.[269]

In keeping with the decisions of the two committees in favor of integration of problematic children within the framework of youth villages, along with their peers, Dr. Berachiahu approached Szold with a request to convince the administrators of the Shfeyah and Ben Shemen youth villages to allocate several places every year for hard-to-educate youth. Szold agreed, and approached the Meir Shfeyah Youth Village through the good offices of Dr. Yitzhak-Dov Berkson, head of the Education Department. In her letter, Szold described the part of the Social Welfare Department she headed, in care for neglected, abandoned and delinquent youth, hard-to-educate and retarded children. She explained that in many cases she had become aware that "there is no cure for children except to place them in the proper educational facilities or put them in private homes."[270] Dr. Berachiahu — who was also a member of the committee, charged with care of hard-to-educate and delinquent children operating under his Department's auspices — revealed that in recent years he had succeeded in gaining admittance to Shfeyah for children of this kind, particularly hard-to-educate ones — and the results were remarkable, without any effect on the way of things within the institution.[271] Upon Dr. Berachiahu's recommendation, Szold wrote the administration of the Shfeyah Youth Village requesting they set aside al least four places for hard-to-educate children each year, promising that she would recommend only children who "would not cause any disturbance to set arrangements," stressing: "A positive response from the institution will serve as an example for additional institutions and in this manner, it will be possible to place an honest number of hard-to-educate children annually."[272]

Overall, this solution was of marginal value, of course, since the number of children in need of help was tremendous, and Dr. Berachiahu did not succeed in placing all within suitable educational frameworks. Consequently, he suggested that Szold prepare a list of institutions, workshops, places of employment and foster families in the city and rural communities that were prepared to come to the assistance of the Department, when necessary, and accept neglected and hard-to-educate children into their care. Szold did her best to find suitable solutions to these problems, but came to the conclusion that the primary difficulty was financial, noting: "Care of a child requires many resources…and as long as we lack adequate resources, it seems to me we won't be able to succeed in our project."[273]

Szold's attitude angered Dr. Berachiahu, for throughout the entire period of his term of office he had engaged in mobilization of funding for his Department and knew that without assistance from suitable institutions, he could not bring about the rehabilitation of hard-to-educate children. Therefore he responded pointedly, saying:

> We have never had enough financial resources, for where is the country in the world that has sufficient means to place all the neglected and retarded children in facilities and so forth? Secondly, and this is the main thing, it's possible today to work and bring benefit to a limited number of children more or less, and to aspire and hope that in the future we will succeed in our endeavor.[274]

Dr. Berachiahu emphatically called upon Szold to approach organizations such as the *Noar Haoved* — the Labor Zionist Youth Movement — and the Workers' Federation of the Social Welfare Committee to prepare a list of owners of workshops, and kibbutz or *moshav* communities willing to employ youths aged 12–18. He reasoned:

> …There is no doubt that we will be able to find people that will take these youngsters to their homes, for they will bring [the employers] benefit through their work. If we can place 10 children a year and make them into social human beings in place of being delinquent, we have done something important and we may aspire to do more.[275]

Dr. Berachiahu closed on an optimistic note:

> We are only at the beginning of our work, and I cannot in any way agree to despair, because despair and leaving the children on their own are surely an unforgivable sin. And it's the Social Welfare Department's duty to encourage the Yishuv regarding this neglected public work.[276]

Moreover, Dr. Berachiahu called upon Szold to convene an immediate meeting of the Medical Committee and invite specialists with experience working with hard-to-educate children to participate and present their opinions — a key to mobilizing support and applying public pressure.[277]

In the end, Szold responded positively to Dr. Berachiahu's request, approached the governing committee of the Meir Shfeyah Youth Village requesting they accept three hard-to-educate children. Two months later, Dr. Berachiahu reported to her that the children who had been recommended had been accepted, and a list had been made of candidates who would be admitted if a place became available during the year. But despite Dr. Berachiahu's ceaseless efforts, many children "for whom maintaining them in the house of the parents was impossible"[278] were still left without an educational solution to their problem, and lacking an alternative were referred to the reformatory in Tul Karem.

Strangely enough, the positive work of Dr. Berachiahu did not receive the blessings and support of the Education Department, who instead even placed obstacles in his way. Dr. Yitzhak-Dov Berkson — director of the Education Department and recipient of Szold's letter regarding integration of hard-to-educate children in the Shfeyah and Ben Shemen youth villages — opposed the idea. He argued that the institutions were not designed for retarded children, only normal children and neglected children "but healthy in body and mind"[279] and that a regular yearly quota of hard-to-educate children would increase their total number within a few years, undoubtedly placing a burden on the villages' work. Szold sent a copy of this letter to Dr. Berachiahu adding that she "found the rationale brought forth in the above letter to be most justified, and I can't, therefore, oppose them."[280]

The problem of rehabilitating problematic children in the educational system continued to bother Dr. Berachiahu. Despite the difficulties in his path, he strove for many years to expand the network of stations designed to serve hard-to-educate children, to open new closed institutions, and to train more youth counselors for these facilities. He was in the habit of saying: "We need money and investments, but these investments will yield great profits. They will give us returns, not in pounds nor shillings, but in the mental health of the young generation."[281]

In historic terms, one can state emphatically that the School Hygiene Department, and Dr. Berachiahu at its head, were pioneers in the establishment of a system for provision of services for mentally disabled schoolchildren — the hard-to-educate, the retarded, the neglected and the delinquent. Under the wing of the School Hygiene Department this problematic juvenile population received, for the first time in their lives, treatment, guidance, counseling and direction in their education from a professionally trained teaching staff, and a team of Department doctors and nurses. Due to Dr. Berachiahu's persistence, and the importance he assigned to rehabilitation of these schoolchildren, mental hygiene evolved and developed as an integral part of the educational infrastructure. This achievement was hallmarked not only by the establishment of institutions for retarded schoolchildren, but also by Consultation Stations designed to diagnose and treat exceptional children — what we term today marginalized groups and children-at-risk — a framework which was adopted and expanded under his direction.

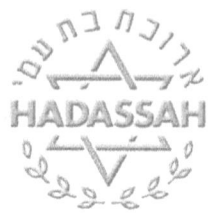

Chapter IV

Mother & Child Health Centers

A. Landmarks in the Development of Treatment of New Mothers & the Struggle with Infant Mortality in Eretz Israel[282]

From the outbreak of the Crimean War between Turkey and Russia in 1953, until the close of the war in the spring of 1856, the link between Russian-Polish Jewry and the Jews of Eretz Israel was severed. Under an edict by Tzar Nicholai I, monetary assistance ceased. As a result of the war, the economic situation of the Yishuv deteriorated and many were left without a source of livelihood and suffered dire famine.

James Finn, the British Consul in Eretz Israel in the years 1845–1863, describes in his memoirs the terrible state into which the residents of Jerusalem were thrown by the war:

> ...The situation of the poor among the Jews at this time, was beyond everything we had known previously. It was said that parents sold their children to Muslims, for this was the only way to save their souls... Small children would cry at night from hunger until they fell asleep...In the terrible year of 1854, we discovered the true situation of the Jewish Quarter. It became clear to us with a clarity we had never seen before, that there were among the Jews in Jerusalem a level of desperate want and poverty that people cannot imagine who had not witnessed the state

*of this wretched People...the level of mortality among poor Jews from
lack of enough food, water and clean air was very large. Now within the
hardships of 1854, it was of a terrible magnitude.*[283]

The British Jewish philanthropist Sir Moses Montefiore (1784–1885)
was the first to come to the aid of the Yishuv. He journeyed through Eretz
Israel a number of times and became active assisting in the establishment
of charitable institutions in various cities, and developing crafts and
industry.[284] Among his activities were the establishment of a medical
clinic and pharmacy, coverage of the salary of the clinic physician Dr.
Shimon Fraenkel, purchase of medicines and the establishment of a fund
to support new mothers.

The Jews of France also responded to the call for help and sent Albert
Cohen — the president of the Federation of Jewish Communities in France
who was also in charge of the Rothschild family's charitable activities —
"to establish constructive and educational undertakings in the country to
extricate the sons of the Yishuv from their distress."[285] Cohen sojourned
in Jerusalem for three weeks, during which time he founded a number of
humanitarian institutions that included a Jewish hospital in Jerusalem on
July 26, 1854 — named after Meir Rothschild, the eldest don of Yaakov
James de Rothschild — and a charitable fund for new mothers and their
infants named after the Baroness Betty de Rothschild. The purpose of the
latter was "to provide mothers and their children with necessary medical
assistance and clothes, and in addition small financial support."[286]

Two years later, Meir Rothschild visited Eretz Israel in order to inspect
institutions and other undertakings established by Albert Cohen. He
expanded funding for the charitable fund designed to support indigent
new mothers and their infants, and set forth a new constitution for the
fund that increased support to cover 14 new mothers a month. Thus, the
fund provided support for a total of 120 new mothers annually by granting
funding to purchase clothing and nutritional needs — stipulating that
Jews of Ashkenazi and Sephardic origin were to be treated "all as equal."[287]
The fund employed two midwives that assisted indigent expectant women
in childbirth.[288]

It should be noted that supporting both Ashkenazi and Sephardic mothers was atypical, as most aid was given by particular communities in the Diaspora for Jews from their own region or religious camp, or earmarked for a particular ethnic group.

In 1872, a special hospital for children, named *Marienstift* (Mary's Foundation), was founded in Jerusalem. The hospital operated for 27 years under the direction of a German Christian physician, Dr. Max Sandreczky. The hospital was non-sectarian and operated under the auspices of the German consulate. The staff included a physician, a male nurse and two female nurses. At the outset, the hospital had only 15 beds, but within a decade its facilities had expanded to hospitalize 200 patients. In its last years of operation the hospital treated some 343 sick children annually with 5,692 hospital days.[289]

In 1890 the *Ezrat Nashim* (Women's Aid) Society was founded in Jerusalem, designed to assist sick women and new mothers in need, prior to and after childbirth. Several years later the *Ezer Yoldot* (Assistance to New Mothers) Society was founded and took upon itself the care of all indigent new mothers. These were the first women's organizations in Eretz Israel to engage in charitable activities that embodied a social welfare role. The tremendous need for assistance to mothers and children stemmed from the fact that in these times, there were no certified midwives or registered nurses in the country. Women were accustomed to giving birth in their homes, "where the mother and newborn lay on the floor, while an old women, dressed in torn and squalid clothing, stood near by."[290] Childbirth took place without proper medical attention or hygienic or sanitary conditions — often endangering the lives of mothers and newborns. Poor hygiene, shortage of water and lack of adequate and proper nutrition led to a high level of infant mortality. Many new mothers did not seek medical assistance or go to hospitals due to ignorance, hindered by superstitions that prompted them to prefer the assistance of local uncertified midwives who had learned their art as apprentices to an older experienced neighborhood midwife or had received their training in the maternity wards opened in the hospitals established in Jerusalem toward the end of the nineteenth century.[291] A midwife came to the woman's house with her belongings and stayed for a number of days to help the new mother and the rest of the family. Only at the beginning of the twentieth century did expert certified midwives who had received their training in Europe begin to settle in Jerusalem.[292]

Itta Yellin wrote in her memoirs in 1940 that the midwife was called only to "well-known families." She wrote of her character: "She was elderly, wise, adroit and clean and with a lot of experience in childbirth, not just among Ashkenazi women but also among Sephardic women, and even the Muslim women had confidence in her."[293]

The midwife served as both nurse and cook. She supervised mother and newborn, laundering and cooking. Care of the newborn was different in those days. Feeding was unstructured, Yellin recalled: "Back then they didn't take notice of the hour or timing of nursing every three or four hours, for when the child began to cry they quickly gave him to his mother to quiet him."[294]

The manner of swaddling was made according to ancient, medieval custom. It was done in this way until well into the nineteenth century:

> *The newborn was wrapped up — prior to being dressed in a gown and shirt, with a narrow bandage around the belly, diapers and a small blanket around half the body and another blanket on the rest of the body together with the hands, with only the face exposed. In this manner the infant was subjugated and diapered in a way that it was possible to hold it without any fear that God forbid one of its organs would be damaged, when it was put in its cradle or taken out. Thus were newborns kept for three to four months like prisoners in shackles.*[295]

Reasons for Infant Mortality

The precarious health and arduous economic straits of the Jews of Jerusalem led to extremely high rates of illness and mortality. Uziel Schmelz, who studied the period, classified a high incidence of illness and death among infants[296] due to unhygienic living conditions and crowding; lack of lighting, fresh air, sewage, accompanied by filth and foul odors; lack of public services for removal of sewage and garbage; collection of water in cisterns insufficient in quantity and quality; malnutrition; insufficient clothing and heating during the winter; widespread disease and epidemics;

the frequency of drought and famine years; and premature marriages that impaired the health and longevity of young mothers and their offspring.

Ch. Sh. Halevi, head of the Hadassah Medical Federation Statistics Department, carried out the first study to examine and analyze one of the most important problems facing the Yishuv from a national-social-welfare standpoint: the problem of infant mortality and its roots. Halevi noted a number of additional factors in his findings:[297]

The age of the mother. Among young mothers (age 18 and under) the rate of infant mortality was above average because the birth weight of these infants was generally lower than the offspring of older mothers.

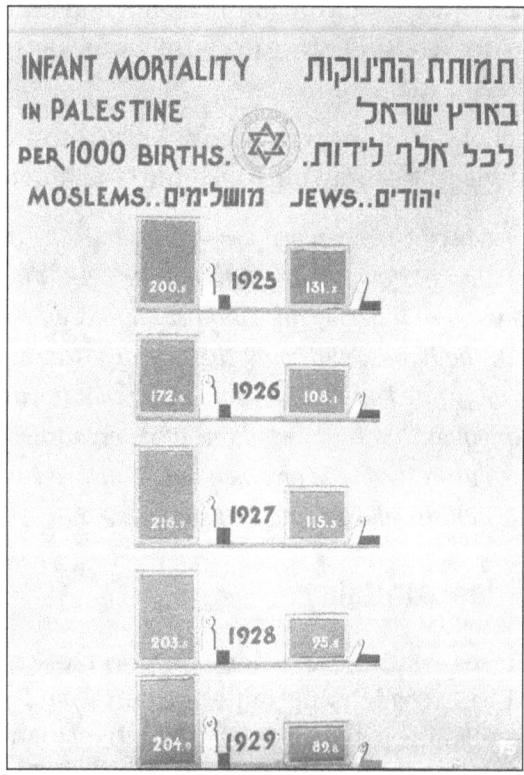

Hadassah Poster- Infant mortality in Eretz Israel per 1000 births, Infant mortality in the Jewish community was much lower that among the Arab community (Donchin-Hadassah Collection).

The large number and frequency of pregnancies that weakened the mother and had a detrimental effect on the infant's ability to survive.

Impoverished living conditions among large families. The mother could not devote herself solely to care of her newborn while she was also responsible for other small children.

Levels of care of the mother and child prior to, during and following childbirth. Lack of care and medical supervision of the newborn — primarily in the first months of life — also had a significant influence on infant mortality.

Infant feeding regimes. Feeding was the first and foremost factor in infant mortality stemming from abdominal and intestinal ailments. It was found that infants who were nursed by their mothers during the entire first year of life were more robust than those who received nutritional substitutes after birth.

Living conditions in general. Primitive conditions — lack of water or sewage systems — aggravated the hygienic straits of large and indigent families, negatively influencing chances of survival among infants.

Climate and weather. Infants born in the summer and fall who were not nursed by their mothers were open to intestinal and abdominal ailments. Infants born in the winter were not adequately protected against diseases stemming from colds, and fell ill with pulmonary ailments.

Only massive, systematic change on behalf of mother and child made it possible to overcome the combined want, ignorance and poverty that especially took a toll on infants. In 1919, Henrietta Szold visited Eretz Israel and was appalled by the poverty and squalor she found among the populations of Jerusalem, Tiberias and Safed — particularly the grave state of hygiene, which Szold felt was the primary factor determining the state of public health. She designed a comprehensive public health program to bring medical aid to mothers and children. The program was launched in 1913 with the assistance of the American Jewish philanthropist Nathan Strauss.

With the outbreak of World War I, Rose Kaplan, one of the two nurses sent to Eretz Israel by Hadassah, left the country. The other nurse, Rachel Landy, continued her mission, together with Dr. Helena Kagan, a

pediatrician who arrived in Eretz Israel from Switzerland in 1914.[298] In
September 1915, when money ran out, Landy was forced to return home
and the clinic was closed. Dr. Kagan continued to extend medical aid in
a clinic she opened in her home near Mea Sha'arim, and even trained
Jewish and Arab girls as nurses in the municipal hospital. To overcome
high infant mortality from malnutrition, Dr. Kagan bought a cow, whose
milk she stored in bottles immersed in clay pots filled with water, giving
the milk to sick babies brought to her clinic. This initiative, however,
solved the problem of only a small number of infants. Dr. Kagan wrote
in her memoirs that the mortality rate after childbirth, primarily from
infection, was horrific:

> Old women uncertified for such [a task] examined the women and
> if they took care to wash their hands, they did so in a basin, in which the
> cleanliness of the water was highly suspect. In addition the towels they
> used served the rest of the family. If the birth did not proceed normally,
> the women poured bottles of oil into the women's uterus. And if in the
> end they nevertheless called for medical aid, the situation [by that time]
> was totally hopeless, and it was already impossible to do anything.[299]

In light of the grievous situation, pediatrician Benno Gruenfelder,
who eventually became the head of the Pediatrics Department of
Hadassah Medical Federation, designed a plan to found a center to care
for pregnant women and infants whose mission was "not just to raise up
a Hebrew generation, but rather a Hebrew generation healthy in body
and spirit."[300] The idea he formulated was eventually to evolve into a
bona fide social welfare treatment center. Dr. Gruenfelder also mentioned
poverty, undernourishment, contagious diseases, lack of hygiene and
lack of knowledge among mothers about nutritional substitutes for breast
milk (called *hazanah melachutit*, "artificial feeding") among the reasons
for high infant mortality. He suggested two primary ways of combating
the situation: Teach mothers how to raise their children and instruct
them about what was required for normal development; and promote a
unified method among doctors and midwives, vis-à-vis care for the health
of mothers and infants.[301]

Dr. Gruenfelder planned to actualize his plans by founding an
"Institute for Growth and Nurturing of Infants" in the Old City, a poor

neighborhood in Jerusalem. In the Institute, a physician who was an expert in infant care would instruct mothers about raising children. If there was need of nutritional substitutes for breast milk, the physician would provide advice about the quality of milk and fortification of cow's milk with other beneficial ingredients.

The physician would be assisted by a nurse, who would instruct the mothers on the importance of maintaining the fundamentals of basic hygiene necessary for the development of their infants such as airing rooms, cleanliness of the house, where to buy fresh milk and from which well to draw water. Dr. Gruenfelder even planned the physical structure of the Institute he envisioned. It was to have two rooms: an anteroom and a room for receiving patients. The doctor would receive the mothers in the inner room, measuring and weighing the children. If conditions in the home were detrimental, the infant would remain at the Institute during the day, in a hygienic environment, and his mother would come to nurse him at regular intervals. Dr. Gruenfelder stressed that:

> ...The first condition for raising the child is nutrition at regular intervals, because irregular feeding is very harmful to the physical development of the child and this is something about which the mothers don't take caution. As soon as the child opens its mouth and cries, they immediately quiet it by feeding, without taking into account at all need or timing.[302]

Dr. Gruenfelder even reported that money to build the Institute was being allocated by a renowned philanthropist and two nurses who had received their training in Europe had already given their consent to work at the facility. Administration of the Institute was turned over to the management of the Federation of Hebrew Women. The outbreak of World War I, however, wrecked preparations, and Dr. Gruenfelder was forced to leave the country, postponing plans for the actualization of his visions.

A fundamental change in this dire situation came only in 1918 with the arrival of the American Zionist Medical Unit in Eretz Israel, sent to assist the Jewish community with health services. The mission found the level of supervision of infants appalling. Decline of the Jewish population due to the war and the character of immigration to Eretz Israel after the war — primarily unmarried women and men — temporarily reduced the number of infants and children in the Yishuv during the years 1919–1922. The devastated state of abject poverty together with an absence of modern rearing techniques, a harsh sub-tropic climate and a high incidence of death among nursing children, all demanded immediate, orderly and systematic supervision of the development of infants — a mission the Unit immediately took upon itself.

B. Care of Pregnant Women and Infants by the American Zionist Medical Unit and the Hebrew Women's Federation

The arrival of the Unit in Eretz Israel marked the beginning of a transitional period — the passage from an era characterized by traditional folk remedies and underdeveloped medical services to an era of modern medicine as we know it. Within the framework of its work in preventive medicine, the Unit's team of doctors and nurses formulated a comprehensive program to assist the population's mothers, infants and children. The Unit's first project in this domain was the opening of the Consultation Station for Mothers & Pregnant Women, in the Old City of Jerusalem — the first of its kind in the country. Soon after its founding, the Station broadened its activities to milk distribution — a project entitled *Tipat Chalav* (A Drop of Milk) that provided pasteurized milk to infants in need. As it became established as an institution, the Station was transformed into a neighborhood health center that attracted mothers and pregnant women from distant neighborhoods.

At the time of the arrival of the Unit, women with a social welfare outlook had already begun organizing themselves to establish various public-spirited projects for those in need, although on a small scale. The harsh economic straits prevailing in Jerusalem, particularly in the Old City — described by the women as "a hub of poverty and distress, where we found child mortality in staggering percentages"[303] — brought the women face-to-face with a population of expectant women, mothers, infants and children who, they said, "reside at the bottom of the heap, as if they had not been touched by the light of the day of developed human beings."[304] The women set for themselves as a central goal to assist their fellow women wherever they may be, particularly during pregnancy and birth, and to provide other women with instruction in care of their offspring. First steps were taken to organize this assistance on a local level — a move that was ultimately transformed into the Hebrew Women's Federation.

The Hebrew Women's Federation

The Hebrew Women's Federation was founded in Jerusalem in 1920 at the initiative of Bat-Sheva Kesselman,[305] prompted by the harsh economic situation prevailing at that time in Eretz Israel. Her goal was "to care for mother and child and raise the status of the women to social and cultural life."[306] Observing the adversity facing woman in the distressed neighborhoods of Jerusalem — particularly pregnant women who gave birth in unhygienic conditions that endangered the woman's health and that of her offspring — Kesselman and other members of the Hebrew Women's Federation found themselves identifying with these other women. Thus, they sought to extend essential aid during pregnancy and birth; to teach them to care for their newborns from the day of birth and to monitor their development and growth; to provide for their material needs; and to teach the women an occupation according to their abilities, and even to help the women find work.[307]

In the beginning, the women organized only on a local basis to address local problems. The first branches were established in Jerusalem (1920), Haifa (1920), Tiberias (1923), Safed (1923), Tel Aviv (1924), and Rechovot (1924) — locations with a high concentration of distressed populations, primarily members of the Jewish community originating from the Middle East and North Africa, who lived under harsh conditions of poor hygiene, malnutrition, lack of education, and were bound to folk superstitions.

During the Purim holiday in March 1924, the first national convention of the Hebrew Women's Federation was held. Henrietta Szold, who agreed to head the organization, defined the overriding objectives of the Hebrew Women's Federation: "The main goal is to organize the women of the country and to amalgamate existing federations into one national federation. Without an umbrella organization it is impossible to do any fruitful work in the country, and it is hard to create ties with women abroad."[308]

The work of the Hebrew Women's Federation was carried out by a central committee composed of three governing bodies: the presidency (the chairwomen, two deputies, and a secretary); the chairwoman of neighborhood communities; and the chairwoman of the committees.

The Federation's endeavors were divided among a number of committees, each focusing on a particular aspect of welfare activity designed to enhance the wellbeing of women and children.

The *Mother Committee* was responsible for women during pregnancy and in the first days after childbirth. The committee's role was to locate pregnant women in the community and convince them to receive medical supervision from Hadassah physicians at the Rothschild-Jerusalem Hospital. Members of the committee visited the homes of expectant women, evaluated their material circumstances, and decided accordingly whether to grant the mother material assistance. If home hygiene was inadequate, they arranged for the women to give birth in a hospital, rather than at home, as was customary in those days.

The *Child Committee* was responsible for women following childbirth, and for care of the newborn and instructing the women in her role as a new mother. The committee formulated the idea of establishing infant care stations where the mother could receive professional advice from doctors and nurses, and the infants would be under ongoing medical supervision from birth until the age of two. Committee members were assigned responsibility for "propagandizing" among mothers to cajole and convince them to visit the station that was established for this purpose in the Old City. This was one of the most difficult missions with which the Hebrew Women's Federation had to cope; it was difficult to convince the women in the in Old City to bring their *healthy* babies to be checked weekly. Moreover, committee officials had to battle superstitions that were common among the mothers,[309] such as reluctance to permit their babies to be weighed for fear of the evil eye. Committee members assisted at the station as doctors and nurses conducted their examinations and helped register infants. They carried out house visits and provided material assistance to the needy. They distributed milk to infants during the first year of life in cases where mothers were unable to nurse due to illness or insufficient supply of breast milk. Children in their second year received canned milk on doctor's orders.

The *Infants' House Committee* cared for foundlings and orphaned infants and babies that could not be raised in the home due to various reasons, such as illness of the mother, living conditions, economic distress, etc. Efforts by committee members brought about establishment of a live-in nursery (Infant House, or *Beit Tinokot* in Hebrew), which opened in 1924. The first of its kind in Eretz Israel, Hadassah provided medical care to the facility. In most cases, the children stayed at the institution until the age of two, and only then were returned to their parents' home.[310]

The *Sewing Committee* was responsible for allocation of packages of diapers for needy infants; some of the packages were received from Hadassah, and some were sewn by committee members. In time, committee members did not merely distribute clothing, but began developing educational aspects of their mission — teaching mothers to sew their children's clothing themselves — in keeping with hygienic requirements and climatic conditions in the country. For this purpose, "sewing centers" were established in a number of Mother & Child Health Centers, where pregnant women gathered together to sew clothing for their newborns under instruction from experienced committee members. The mothers purchased material from the sewing center at a nominal price, in order not to accustom them to take charity.

The *Cultural Committee* initiated classes to teach Hebrew and organized lectures for women in poor neighborhoods on educational and social subjects. The committee took it upon itself to extricate Jewish children from Christian mission schools and place them in Hebrew (i.e., Jewish) schools. Committee members also organized evening classes for 13- to 14-year-old girls who worked during the day and thus were unable to attend regular school.

The *Kindergarten Committee*, thanks to the efforts of its members, was able to mobilize enough funding to permit opening a kindergarten in the Old City in 1924 for 80 children, and a second kindergarten in the Shimon Tzedek neighborhood of Jerusalem for 50 children.[311]

In its educational-cultural endeavors, the Hebrew Women's Federation collaborated with the Unit. The two bodies played a central role in the operation of Mother & Child Health Centers. The Unit supplied medical services and the Hebrew Women's Federation administered social welfare work and participated in the operation of *Tipat Chalav* (A Drop of Milk) stations, with milk pasteurized under Hadassah supervision.

In 1921, the two bodies formulated a joint agreement as to the role of each within the framework of the organization of welfare activities for mothers and children. The plan for cooperation between the Hebrew Women's Federation and the Unit called for concentrating on needy Jewish mothers, reserving for a later stage the broadening of operations to encompass care for nursing children and newborns. Work was divided into three areas: prenatal care of expectant women, assistance in childbirth and post-delivery care.

Prenatal Care of Pregnant Women

Care of expectant women included both material and medical assistance. The Hebrew Women's Federation located pregnant women in poor neighborhoods, mainly in Jerusalem, and extended economic-material aid that included instruction in preparation of supplies necessary for the impending birth and post-delivery care, such as sheets and underclothing for mother and child. Particularly needy women received this material assistance gratis. Medical care of the women began in the sixth month of pregnancy and included medical examinations carried out in the maternity ward of the Rothschild-Hadassah Hospital. Pregnant women remained under the medical supervision of Unit physicians until delivery of their offspring.

It was agreed that receipt of medical care would be a precondition for receipt of material care — that is to say, pregnant women who came to be examined regularly and agreed to receive full prenatal care, would receive financial assistance in the form of money and medications. The Unit adopted this strict stipulation despite "the impression created of [being] a despotic practice."[312] The Unit was motivated by the desire to forestall cases of difficult deliveries and to maintain the health of mother and newborn. Indeed, experience showed that among 75% of all Jewish births in Jerusalem that were cared for by the Unit, there was almost no opposition to examinations or prenatal care among Jewish women.[313]

Prenatal care was provided by obstetricians and not by general practitioners or midwives. At the time of registration with the local committee of the Hebrew Women's Federation, each pregnant woman was given a special card on which her family and economic status were registered. This data was used to determine the type of assistance that would be rendered by the Unit — whether the woman would give birth in the hospital or at home with a midwife in attendance, and whether assistance would be granted gratis or entail payment for services. The Unit's maternity ward cared for some 30 deliveries a month — 360 annually. The new mothers received initial instructions on care for their newborns while still in the hospital. The ward also served as makeshift "mothers' instruction stations," providing elementary guidance on childcare and health maintenance.[314]

At the end of 1922, the delegated heads of Hadassah in Eretz Israel and the leaders of the Hebrew Women's Federation decided that pregnant women would be accepted by the maternity ward of the Rothschild-Hadassah Hospital regardless of financial status, as long as there was a free bed. If two women arrived, however, one needy and the other affluent, the needy woman would be admitted. If one was needy and the other "a pathological case," the latter would receive preferential treatment. If a needy women would have to deliver her offspring at home with the aid of a midwife, the Hebrew Women's Federation would assist her as much as possible with the delivery. Hadassah adopted a payment system in medical services for maternity cases that classified women into five groupings according to family income: The first received free care, the last paid the full rate prevailing in private facilities, and the others paid fees based on a graduated scale according to the individual's economic status.[315]

Assistance in Delivery

The Hebrew Women's Federation assisted women in labor to get to the hospital or called a midwife to the house. Due to the limited capacity of the maternity ward in the Rothschild-Hadassah Hospital, there were women who gave birth in their homes, assisted by one of the Unit's midwives. Those referred for hospital deliveries were cases of difficult labor and particularly poverty-stricken women whose home conditions were not suitable for home deliveries. Members of the Federation were aware of such cases, and instructed each expectant woman what to do. In home delivers, one of the Federation women was sent to the home of women in labor to help the midwife where needed "without her interfering, of course, in [the midwife's] professional task."[316] Assistance included providing hot water, heating and caring for other children in the home, purchasing food and providing for all the needs of the family.

Postnatal Care

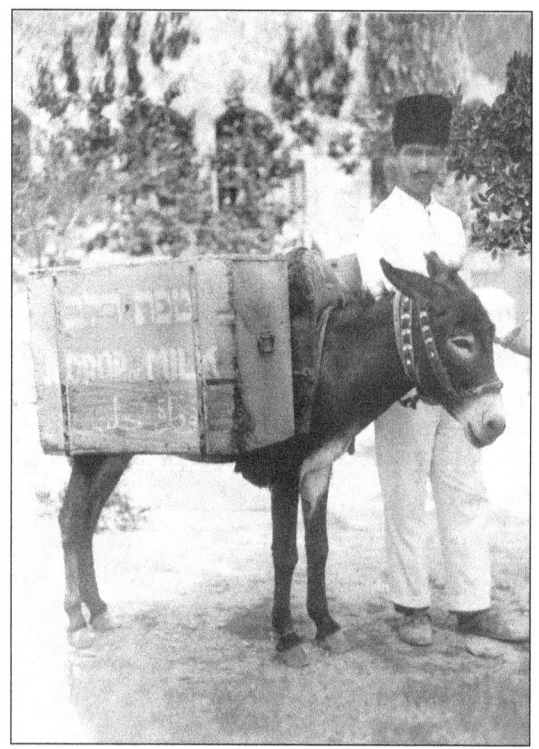

The Donkey Milk Express (Courtesy of Hadassah Archives, NY).

Postnatal aid extended by the Hebrew Women's Federation lasted four weeks. During the first ten days after delivery, assistance was ongoing — including attending to all domestic needs and ensuring that the midwife visited the new mother daily. After the first ten days, the new mother remained under the supervision of Federation women for a total of four weeks.

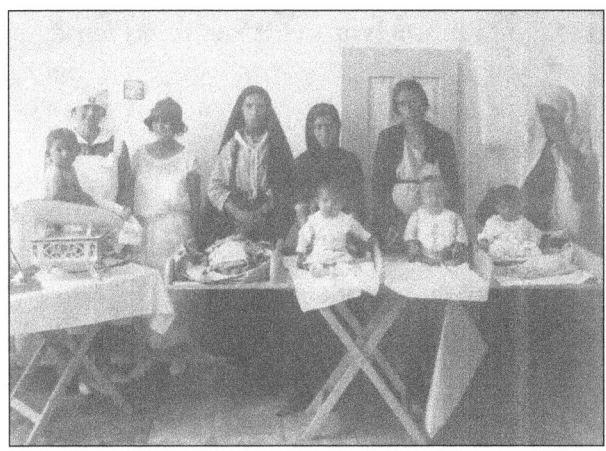

Maternal and child welfare stations for Arab women; Hadassah provided equal services for pregnant women and children among the Arab community, early 1920s (Donchin-Hadassah Collection).

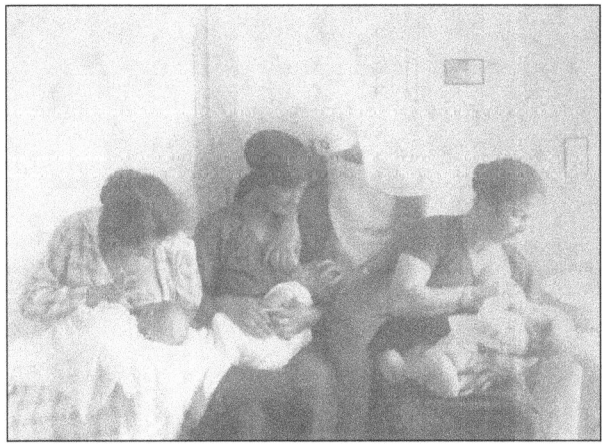

Mothers breast feeding support meeting (Donchin-Hadassah Collection).

The work of the Unit among pregnant women, mothers and children brought about a fundamental change in public attitudes toward provision of preventive medical services to pregnant women, mothers and newborns. In terms of prevailing concepts of the times, the change was truly revolutionary, for until the arrival of the Unit in Eretz Israel, pregnant women, new mothers and children received no care or medical attention whatsoever. With the assistance of the Hebrew Women's Federation, the Unit brought about a significant change in attitudes, providing medical services, instruction and guidance to mothers on caring for and raising their children. Within the framework of preventive medicine, the Unit formulated a comprehensive health plan that began with the establishment of a "consultation station for mothers and pregnant women" that evolved into a model for Mother & Child Health Centers that were later successfully established throughout the country.

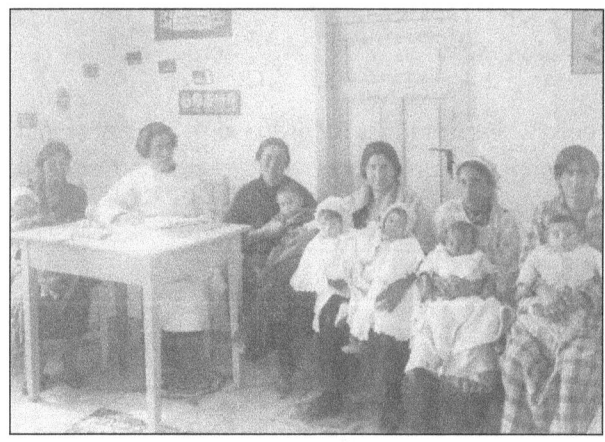

Waiting for the weekly visit in the Tipat Chalav station, 1930s
(Donchin-Hadassah Collection).

C. The Hadassah Health Centers in Jerusalem: A Model for Mother & Child Health Centers

The first Hadassah Health Center in Eretz Israel was opened in July 1921 in the Old City of Jerusalem. The goal was "to educate and to raise the life of the masses to a certain cultural level in those places where neglect and slovenliness has rooted itself."[317] The Center was designed to fulfill three functions: provide guidance to pregnant women; provide guidance and advice to mothers on care of their infants; and prepare and distribute pasteurized milk to infants in need through *Tipat Chalav.*

Beginnings

In the beginning, the Center operated under makeshift conditions. Bertha Landsman, who began her work in Eretz Israel in the pediatrics department of the Rothschild-Hadassah Hospital, became acutely cognizant of the high infant mortality rate in the Old City of Jerusalem during the first year of life. She came to the conclusion that weighty medical forces should be focused on reducing infant mortality. To do so, Landsman established a station to care for nursing babies, modeled after Mother & Child Stations established under the patronage of Nathan Straus in New York, where she had been employed prior to immigrating to Eretz Israel. To forward this goal, Landsman rented a residential structure in the Old City with two rooms and a kitchen. While the house was "ramshackle and half-gloomy and the walls covered with moisture and mildew,"[318] she rented it nevertheless, in order to prove to local residents that with willpower and attention, the neglected structure could be turned into "a pearl."

The house was whitewashed and equipped "in the utmost simplicity, but pleasantly and tastefully furnished,"[319] and all furniture was painted light blue. The facility was organized thus: One room was turned into a receiving room for Dr. Helena Kagan, the volunteer physician. The room was equipped with a dividing screen, a desk upon which a scale for weighing babies was placed, the other half serving as a place where babies could be laid down. A desk shaped like a cabinet served as an examination table. The second room, which served as a waiting room for the mothers, was decorated with instructional posters and a table that served as a "display," demonstrating equipment "of hygienic value" such as "methods of fighting flies, a 'cooler,' and an infant cradle made out of a cardboard carton, and baby clothes."[320] The display was changed from time to time and served as a source of instruction for the mothers.

The kitchen was converted into a milk station. Supplied with primitive equipment for pasteurizing milk, the kitchen became a milk distribution station for babies in need. The milk project was labeled *Tipat Chalav*. Over time, other titles for the facility — "Health Center," "Consultation Center for Mothers & Pregnant Women," "Nursing Babies Care Station," and so forth — were gradually dropped and the name *Tipat Chalav* became associated with the institution in the public mind and eventually was officially adopted as the name and "address" for a broad spectrum of mother and child functions and services, beyond milk distribution. The name is still in use today.

On the second floor of the house, Hadassah established an eye clinic and general clinic for the convenience of Old City residents. Over time the facility was transformed into a community health center. Clinic hours were arranged for optimal isolation; a pediatrician received babies for examination in the morning and an ophthalmologist received patients with trachoma and other diseases in the afternoon, keeping contact between patients on the first and second floors to a minimum.

Once the Health Center was organized and running, the nurses were surprised to find that the number of mothers using the Center's services was low, forcing the organizers "to go out onto the streets."[321] Nurses and volunteers from the Hebrew Women's Federation canvassed the neighborhood to convince mothers to come to the Health Center to receive guidance and advice on raising their children. They "hunted for every expectant woman encountered in the streets, in the alleys or elsewhere."[322] The residents, however, stood firm in their refusal to come to the Health Center, primarily due to superstition and objection to any outside interference of modernity in their traditional way of life and refusal to accept guidance from young, single nurses who had never given birth themselves and therefore were considered unequipped to give advice. As previously mentioned, the women objected to weighing and measuring their infants for fear of the evil eye, and rejected calls to swaddle their babies in a less restrictive manner than the way they had learned from their own mothers and grandmothers in which extremities were tightly bound "to maintain the body in a good position."[323] When the nurses conducted home visits, they found babies diapered and wrapped up like mummies that looked more like packages ready to be posted than living beings. The children's eyes were moist from the smoke of coals in the cook stove. Windows were closed to prevent entrance of "evil spirits" and when women did not have sufficient breast milk, they fed their babies unpasteurized goat's milk.[324]

To encourage mothers to visit the Health Center and break their resistance, it was necessary to promise material assistance. The nurses told the mothers that they would receive gratis all the baby's needs — diapers, clothing, bathing equipment and pasteurized milk — if they would go to give birth in the Rothschild-Hadassah Hospital, and come to the Health Center after childbirth with their infants for continued treatment and instruction in the care of their babies. Only after the nurses succeeded in gaining the trust of the mothers and convincing them that they could enhance the health of their children did regular visits become routine.[325]

In August 1921, a second *Tipat Chalav* station was established in a wooden cottage built in the courtyard of the Rothschild-Hadassah Hospital. The station provided guidance to mothers and served as a milk distribution point for children in the New City of Jerusalem, in the western part of the city beyond the Old City walls. During its first year of operation, over 700 infants were registered at the two *Tipat Chalav* stations. However, only half the newborns were actually brought to the stations, even after nurses made house visits and promised material assistance to convince the mothers to come.

Nevertheless, the milk distribution station adjacent to the hospital registered a steady rise in visits during its first year of operation in 1922:[326] 26 in January, 41 in February, 48 in March, and 68 in April. In light of the rise in attendance, Landsman wrote Szold calling for expansion of the staff so all children would receive the best medical-hygienic care possible. A joint meeting was convened to organize the work of the two *Tipat Chalav* stations. In attendance were Dr. Rubinow, Dr. Kagan, Landsman and Szold. At the conclusion, the following decisions were made: Present staffing for the two Health Centers — capable of providing services for a maximum of 200 children — was insufficient. Therefore, a nurse-intern would be appointed to assist Landsman in preparing milk formulas, providing guidance to mothers, and conducting home visits. Milk would be provided only to babies brought regularly on a weekly basis to one of the two consultation stations and only these babies would be visited at home by Hadassah nurses. Mothers interested in whole milk for their children in addition to the milk provided by the station could receive the milk on their own at points were milk was sold — at regular prices.[327]

In July 1923, the Hebrew Women's Federation planned to open a third Health Center in a kindergarten in the Machaneh Yehuda neighborhood of West Jerusalem that would serve as a milk distribution point and provide weekly consultation for mothers — including examinations by a pediatrician. However, opening of the Center became a source of fierce disagreement between Hadassah and the Hebrew Women's Federation over payment of nurses' salaries.

Hadassah, suffering from financial problems of its own, declined to shoulder the economic burden. Therefore Bat-Sheva Kesselman "threatened" Szold that if Hadassah would not fulfill the request and pay the salary of the nurse, as president of the Hebrew Women's Federation Kesselman would accept an offer from WIZO (Women's International Zionist Organization) to appoint a nurse from among the "rival" Jewish women's organization, in order to inaugurate the new Center. Hadassah management could not accept such a move, for the Health Centers established by Hadassah in Jerusalem were a pioneering operation for mothers and children that were viewed by Hadassah as a future model for similar centers throughout the country. Consequently, Hadassah clarified that WIZO and the Hebrew Women's Federation would not be allowed "to make inroads" into this area of work, although the latter extended aid and volunteer support to Hadassah. Consequently, the new Health Center was opened under the administration of Hadassah — through donations sent by women's groups in Brooklyn and American Jewish philanthropist Nathan Straus, involving local women from the Hebrew Women's Federation in social welfare activities.[328]

Under the influence of their Jewish neighbors, Arab women — Muslim and Christian — also began to seek guidance at the Health Center in the Old City. In response, in 1923 an Arabic-speaking nurse was appointed to work solely with Arab mothers. Her salary was paid by Lina and Nathan Straus; one day a week was scheduled for guidance for these women. As the number of Arab women approaching the Center grew, plans were drawn up to register 100 women as a precondition for opening a Health Center in an Arab neighborhood.

Indeed, in 1924 a Health Center was inaugurated adjacent to the Nablus Gate of the Old City in the Arab Quarter, designed to serve mothers and children among the Arab population. Hadassah management rented a suitable structure and equipped it with all necessary equipment. The nurse who worked in this Center had been trained in public nursing at Hadassah's nursing school. Unlike women at the three Jewish Health Centers, women at the new Center received medical assistance gratis from Dr. Caspari — director of the Hadassah Health Centers in Jerusalem until 1926. Afterwards, medical assistance was provided by Dr. Benno Gruenfelder, Hadassah's head physician for pediatrics and supervisor of Hadassah Health Centers. In addition to Jewish doctors, for a period of time Arab doctors also worked on a volunteer basis in the new Center. The first to do so was Dr. Hadad, who worked on a volunteer basis at the Center between 1924 and September 1925. Dr. Dajani took over during the last quarter of 1926 and was subsequently relieved by Dr. Hussein Abu Said, who had volunteered during the first months of 1926. From mid-1926 until the closure of Nablus Gate Health Center in April 1928 — due to redundancy of health services in the neighborhood following the establishment of similar government-sponsored services — Dr. Gruenfelder worked on a volunteer basis at the Arab clinic.[329]

Health Center Operation Methods

Hadassah was responsible for the medical-informative aspects of work at the Health Centers, while the Hebrew Women's Federation ran the social welfare and administrative side of operations including registration of new mothers and infants; writing of monthly reports; mobilization of volunteers to help out at the centers; and administering payment for milk by mothers, which was graduated according to the economic status of the family. Expenditures were also divided between the two bodies: Hadassah paid the rent, appointed doctors and registered nurses and nurse-interns and paid their salaries, including the salaries of the person who delivered the milk and the janitor; the Hebrew Women's Federation paid for the milk.

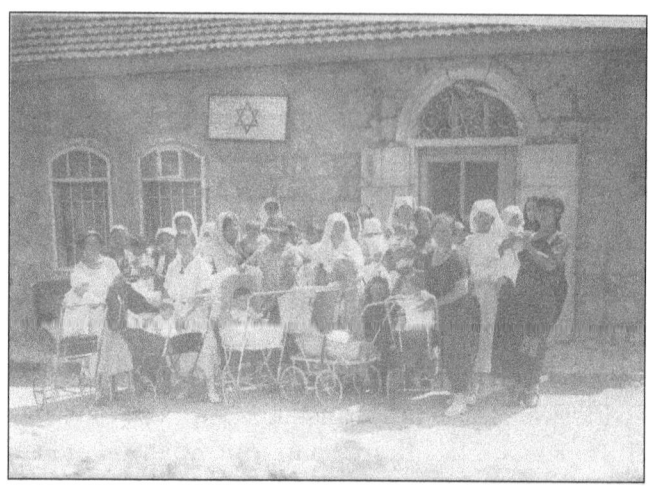

*Maternal and child welfare center Tipat Chalav
Station 1930s (Donchin-Hadassah Collection).*

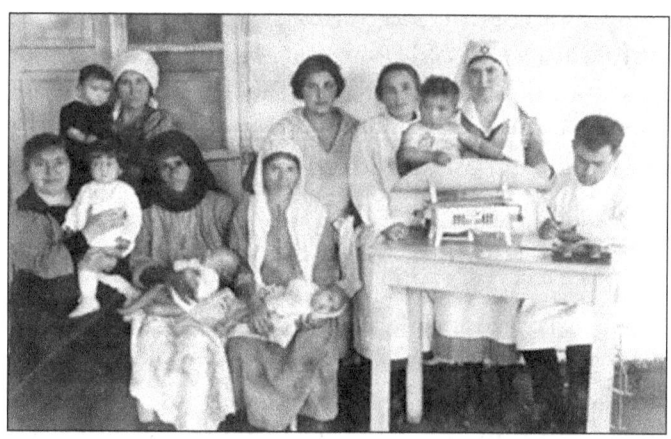

*Hadassah maternal and child welfare center Tipat Chalav for Arab mothers
in old city Jerusalem 1920-1930s (Donchin-Hadassah Collection).*

On the day consultations were conducted, some 60–70 mothers
visited the clinic with their children. Women's Federation volunteers
received them in the anteroom, ensuring each would receive timely,

satisfactory service. The volunteers dealt with all administrative duties, thus freeing the nurse to assist the doctor. The volunteer prepared the nursing child's chart and called each mother in turn into the weighing room. The nurse–intern weighed the baby and updated its personal chart. According to the child's development and weight, it was decided whether the child should be examined by the doctor (if the child was not scheduled for a regular checkup). With the assistance of the chief nurse, the doctor examined the child, aided by the child's personal chart. The mother received guidance and instruction on the care of her baby, its development and nutrition. Babies in need received pasteurized milk from another Hebrew Women's Federation volunteer. The volunteers were assigned an additional mission: to locate all nursing babies in the neighborhood under the age of 12 months and convince mothers to bring their children to the Health Center to receive instruction and care, and conduct follow-up to determine whether the mothers had, in fact, shown up at the clinic.[330]

Tipat Chalav Operation Methods

Tipat Chalav stations constituted a department within the Health Centers and were organized by nurses who were graduates of Hadassah's nursing school, together with nursing interns. The station operation was located in the Health Center's kitchen, and equipped to pasteurize the milk. A *Tipat Chalav* Committee of Hebrew Women's Federation members was responsible for administration, and volunteers together with Hadassah nurses collaborated in its operation.

The nurses learned to prepare milk formulas and measured feedings in bottles according to the individual needs of the infant. Fresh milk was brought daily to the station from the dairy in Kiryat Anavim, a kibbutz located just outside Jerusalem. A sanitation physician[331] from the Rothschild-Hadassah Hospital instructed dairy personnel how to maintain a hygienic dairy farm in regards to both cows and milk. After milking, the raw milk was stored in containers sterilized by the nurses the previous day. Milk samples were sent to the hospital bacteriology laboratory. After the milk passed laboratory inspection, the milk was pasteurized. The process included straining the milk to remove any foreign objects or other material that might contaminate the milk, then heating the milk to just under the boiling point. The hot milk was then quickly immersed in a tub of ice water to rapidly reduce its temperature and poured into sterilized bottles. The result was the first pasteurized milk in Eretz Israel, perhaps even the first in the entire Middle East.

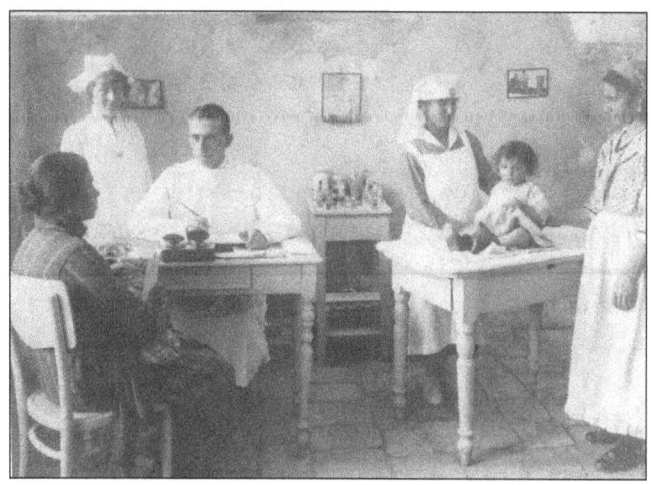

Inside the Tipat Chalav station, weekly visit for child development that was included doctor checkup and nurse follow-up of the child development (especially the weight). Tipat Chalav station for Arabs mothers in the Old City of Jerusalem 1920-1930s (Donchin-Hadassah Collection).

Flora Soloman — who helped equip the milk kitchen and donated funding for allocation of milk and was the wife of Harold Solomon, head of the Mandatory government's Department of Trade and Industry — headed a staff of volunteers who poured the milk into sterilized bottles and distributed it to mothers in need who came to the Health Center. Word spread and mothers from the Old City and beyond began coming to the Center to buy milk "that doesn't rapidly deteriorate."[332] Nevertheless, many mothers were hesitant to come, so Bertha Landsman decided to bring the milk to the mothers. In this manner, what came to be dubbed the "Donkey Milk Express" was founded. The names of the children were written on the bottles and stored inside two crates with the words *"Tipat Chalav"* stenciled on the exterior in Hebrew, English and Arabic. The crates were loaded on the back of a donkey that made its way from the Health Center in the Old City to the Health Center adjacent to Rothschild-Hadassah Hospital where the mothers waited. Volunteers from the Hebrew Women's Federation distributed the pasteurized milk. The mothers paid a nominal price for the milk, except for destitute mothers who received the milk totally free of charge. Once the milk program was well established, Landsman launched the educational program she had envisioned — providing advice to mothers on proper nutrition.

In July 1925, an agreement was signed between Hadassah Medical Federation and the *Tipat Chalav* Committee of the Hebrew Women's Federation in Jerusalem regarding administration of the milk kitchen. The agreement stated that the committee would be responsible for the milk kitchen's budget — 30 Eretz Israel pounds a month (25 donated by Flora Soloman and 5 donated by the Hebrew Women's Federation). The funds were earmarked for expenses required to prepare the milk such as nursing bottles, ice, kerosene, sugar, cost of transporting the milk, writing materials and so forth. Hadassah Medical Federation was to administer and supervise the milk kitchen, pay the rent and water bill, appoint staff (nurse supervisor, nurse-intern, janitor and milk delivery person), and carry out inspections of the dairy farm and bacteriological tests in the lab. Strict adherence to hygiene and sanitation prevented contamination.[333]

According to the agreement, a new arrangement was initiated to administer *Tipat Chalav* stations. A "Unified Committee" was formed, composed of three delegates from the Hadassah Medical Federation and three delegates from the Hebrew Women's Federation *Tipat Chalav* Committee. The first members of the Unified Committee were: Dr. Bleustone, director of the Hadassah Medical Federation; Bertha Landsman, head nurse of the Public Medicine Department; and Dr. Benno Gruenfelder, head physician of the Department for Care of Nursing Children. The delegates appointed by the *Tipat Chalav* Committee included the pediatrician Dr. Helena Kagan and two lay members of the Hebrew Women's Federation. Thus, *Tipat Chalav* received official recognition as a Hadassah institution, working in collaboration with the Hebrew Women's Federation — a joint endeavor reflected in the wording emblazoned on *Tipat Chalav* signs.[334]

Conclusion

The first three Hadassah Health Centers, established in Jerusalem — which historically constituted a representative model for other centers subsequently established around the country — were eventually closed or transferred to other neighborhoods. The first, established in the Old City in 1921, operated until 1935, when it was closed and transformed into a learning center for nurses. At Dr. Yasski's suggestion, Hadassah management decided that the Old City Health Center would become a branch of the organization's nursing school, serving as a learning center in public medicine under Hadassah management. In keeping with this decision, in September 1935, what historically constituted the first Health Center in Eretz Israel became a separate entity, directly linked to the school of nursing. Nursing interns and registered nurses specializing in public medicine worked in the station, providing guidance and instruction to families in the Old City.[335] The second Health Center that operated in the courtyard of the Rothschild-Hadassah Hospital was closed as the hospital expanded, and was transferred to the premises of the Straus Health Center. The third Center, opened near the Nebulas Gate of the Old City in 1924, was closed in April 1928, following the inauguration of two nearby stations to treat pregnant women and nursing babies launched under Mandatory government sponsorship, causing Hadassah management to realize that its own Center was redundant. To prevent waste of resources, the Center was transferred from the Nebulas Gate to another Jerusalem neighborhood badly in need of such services — Givat Shaul in the western part of the city. Subsequently, more and more Health Centers were established in Jerusalem. The program broadened into Mother & Child Health Centers that included comprehensive health programs for guiding pregnant women and mothers in the care of their offspring — a model for all Health Centers established by Hadassah throughout the country.

D. Mother & Child Health Centers in Haifa, Safed, Tiberias and Tel Aviv

Health Centers for treating infants and pregnant women were established "to give advice, instruction and demonstration lessons in health practices"[336] — operations that were carried out throughout the country on an almost identical basis. Each center was established in a three-room apartment, furnished simply in the same model and color. One room was transformed into a waiting room, the second an infant weighing room, and the third a doctor's and nurses' office. All centers were administered by registered nurses assisted by practical nurses. Medical care administered by a volunteer physician — working under the supervision of Hadassah's pediatrics specialist in Eretz Israel — was provided twice a week for infants and once a week for pregnant women.[337]

Tipat Chalav stations were established adjacent to the Health Centers in Jerusalem, Tiberias and Haifa. Operating through donations, the centers prepared pasteurized milk with the help of Hebrew Women's Federation volunteers, for transfer to other stations in their vicinity. Hadassah covered the cost of supervising the dairy farms and bacteriological tests.

Morning hours at the centers were devoted to visits by mothers with children up to the age of four, designed to provide advice on care and nutrition. Supervision of infants was not limited to visits to the centers; care was augmented by home visits by the nurses in order to assess socioeconomic conditions in the home and to extend assistance where needed. The nurses gave weekly lectures to mothers and pregnant women, and conducted weekly lessons on how to cook food suitable for infants and children, such as making gruel and vegetable soup. In a number of centers, a sewing center was even organized where mothers were taught to sew diapers and children's clothes.

Records kept at the time by Bertha Landsman reflect the growth and development of the Health Centers between the years 1922–1926:

Expansion of Infant Welfare and Prenatal Work in Health Centers [338]

Year	Number of Centers	Number of Children	Home Visits
1922	2	357	552
1923	3	584	876
1924	6	781	9,853
1925	9	926	10,261
1926	13	1,628	N/N

The Haifa Health Center

The Hebrew Women's Federation for Mothers and Child Aid was founded in Haifa in August 1922 with the goal of providing "healthy" food to mothers and children, particularly among immigrants who were exposed to high mortality due to malnutrition. Their first mission was to establish a *Tipat Chalav* milk distribution station along the lines of the station operating in the Old City in Jerusalem. Yehudit Katinka, chairperson of the Hebrew Women's Federation, turned to Henrietta Szold requesting that a nurse with expertise in preparation of pasteurized milk for infants be sent to Haifa to provide instruction and assistance in establishing a Health Center.

Szold praised the initiative but was unable to send a nurse as requested due to Hadassah's difficult financial straits at the time. In order not to turn the women volunteers away entirely, Szold suggested a preliminary plan of action: The nurses would go out among the homes of residents and instruct mothers on an individual basis "how to refine milk in their homes by the Pasteur method";[339] Hadassah would supervise the dairy farm, and the milk would be tested in the lab of the Hadassah Hospital in Haifa; Dr. B. Nissenboym, a pediatrician at Hadassah Hospital in Haifa, would instruct the nurses; a nurse from Haifa would be sent to Jerusalem to learn Hadassah work methods from Landsman, who had opened the first Health Center in Jerusalem.

The Haifa branch of the Hebrew Women's Federation was disappointed with Szold's response, explaining that the suggestions were not applicable in Haifa, for the mothers lived a destitute existence under harsh living conditions in shacks and tents and had no way of preparing milk properly. There was apprehension that a delay in establishing a *Tipat Chalav* station would curb the growth of the organization's work. Faced with a sense that there were expectations among Haifa residents "of a concrete project from our association,"[340] the women did not wait for Hadassah assistance, but rather rented a building with the help of a loan and opened a *Tipat Chalav* station. Nurse Tzipora Ashkenazi-Azulai, a graduate of the Hadassah nursing school, was sent to Jerusalem to learn the work of the Health Centers firsthand.

In the meantime, construction of a Health Center in the Hadar neighborhood of Haifa — one of the newly constructed Jewish neighborhoods on the slopes of Mt. Carmel above the lower city on the bay — was begun, supported by the French Committee for Care of Nursing Babies[341] and the Hebrew Women's Federation. Extra support was provided through mobilization of philanthropic donations and collection of money from the public through the organization of dance balls. Although construction took longer than expected, the Center was opened on July 6, 1923.[342] The Center had four rooms, but opened with only one unit — a station for care of nursing babies. The second unit, a *Tipat Chalav* station, was inaugurated only six months later. Distribution of milk was conducted in return for nominal payment — "of course, only a few cents" — and preparation and allocation of formula was carried out by the nurses on the Sabbath, as well.

Establishment, maintenance and operation of the Health Center was conducted jointly by three bodies: The French Committee participated in building costs and paid the salaries of the two nurses; the Hebrew Women's Federation paid for the milk; and the Hadassah Zionist Women's Federation paid the physician's salary, took responsibility for the inspection of the dairy farm and bacteriological tests of the milk, and supplied medications to the Center and oversaw the hospitalization of children.[343]

The opening of the Center was a source of both excitement and suspicion, even evoking opposition in some quarters. Mothers and expectant women did not rush to seek the Center's services. From the outset, the Center faced numerous problems:

Similar to the situation in Jerusalem, a low attendance rate among pregnant women and mothers prompted the staff to promise material assistance in return for coming to the Center on a regular basis. The head nurse in charge of nursing babies, Ella Lipski, initiated a series of lectures for mothers. At first attendance was high, but then dropped. Lipski learned that the destitute circumstances of the mothers was the underlying cause, prompting her to comment:

> *...Their spirits were dampened to a point where their minds were not free for such matters, and each one promised me that as soon as her husband received work she would again come to the lessons. Against arguments such as these, it was hard to respond.*[344]

Moreover, severe disputes developed between the French Committee and Hadassah over management of the Center. The French Women's Association objected to Hadassah's participation in the work of the Center. The French demanded they manage the Health Center independently. Attempting to settle the disagreement, Dr. Nachum Shimkin, Hadassah director in Haifa, suggested that the French Committee would run the *Tipat Chalav* station and the station for nursing babies, while Hadassah would open a third unit, solely under Hadassah management, to care for pregnant women. Friction between the two organizations continued until July 1925 when the French Committee announced that it had decided to discontinue its support of "the institution for care of nursing babies and *Tipat Chalav*" due to disagreements with Hadassah.[345] In the wake of withdrawal of French support, a new arrangement was formulated to keep the Center operating: The Hadassah Zionist Women's Federation in America and the Hebrew Women's Federation in Haifa continued their support of the Center, with expenditures covered with the help of the Nathan Straus Foundation's special infant care fund. The Hebrew Women's Federation continued to underwrite the milk kitchen.

A second Health Center in Haifa was opened in the Lower City at the base of Mt. Carmel in October 1925 under the management of Nurse Zelda Goldman. While the Center in the Hadar neighborhood was designed for the Jewish population that lived in newly constructed neighborhoods on the slopes of Mt. Carmel, this second Center targeted a mixed population of Jews and Arabs who populated the older neighborhoods down in the Lower City near the port. Some 900 children a month were treated at the facility in the Lower City and 200–250 home visits were conducted per month by the Center's nurses.

A third Health Center was opened, also in the Lower City of Haifa, on July 14, 1926, on Ard el-Yahud Street, situated in a neighborhood kindergarten. According to an agreement reached with the chairperson of the Haifa Kindergarten Teachers' Association, the kindergarten could be used by the nurses during afternoon hours. A station for nursing babies and guidance for mothers and pregnant women was opened on the premises. Immediately, some 40 mothers with infants registered. The composition of the population was similar to that in the Lower City — Jews of both Oriental and European origin, and both Christian and Muslim Arabs, all living in a mixed neighborhood. Landsman commented that "these were the poorest children in the city, and the mothers were indigent and uncultured."[346]

The protocols and reports of nurses' meetings in Haifa focusing on the health of children in Haifa reveal that circumstances of infants in the Ard el-Yahud neighborhood were the worst. A large percentage of the infants received milk substitute formulas from an early age, due to difficulty the mothers encountered in nursing their babies. During the summer, the situation worsened and many babies fell ill. Due to the infants' poor general conditions, doctors decided to change nutrition, substituting regular milk with buttermilk. Under normal circumstances buttermilk was reserved for particularly weak, underweight infants threatened by serious intestinal problems in the summer months.[347] In August 1933, a hepatitis epidemic broke out among the children of Ard el-Yahud. Infants were brought to the Health Center and fed buttermilk. In particularly hard cases, they were hospitalized. Nevertheless, three babies died.

A fourth Health Center was opened in Haifa in the Neve Shaanan neighborhood on November 14, 1927 — an event celebrated together with residents of the community. The Center — situated in a large two-room furnished and well-kept apartment — served at the outset some 40–50 children a month, while the nurse in charge of the Center, Ahuva Weinstein, carried out 10 to 15 home visits per month.[348]

By 1935, Hadassah Health Centers in Haifa served 1,170 registered children, most of them in the poor neighborhood of the Lower City in Haifa.

Cooperation between Hadassah and Kupat Holim in the Management of Haifa Health Centers

When Kupat Holim began opening Health Centers modeled after the Hadassah Centers, Hadassah director Dr. Yasski and Kupat Holim medical director Dr. Meir concluded that in all cities and settlements where Kupat Holim established Mother & Child Health Centers, Hadassah would transfer all its patients to these centers. Concurrently, Kupat Holim transferred all its members to Hadassah's centers in the villages of Petach Tikva and Rechovot. In Haifa, transfer was delayed due to negotiations between WIZO, Hadassah and Kupat Holim over formulation of a joint program — on both a financial and administrative level — by which all babies in Haifa would be registered and treated on a geographical basis regardless of the affiliation of family or center.

The first joint meeting between Kupat Holim representatives and Hadassah management to lay the groundwork for cooperation was held in May 1926. Dr. Yasski, then deputy director of Hadassah, justified the move, noting: "It is important to amalgamate systems, upon which the success of this field work hangs, doubly important in a small country such as our country."[349]

It was decided to conduct two consultation days in each of the two Health Centers in Haifa. In other words, on one day a Hadassah physician would visit both Centers and provide advice for all babies in the area, and on another day a Kupat Holim physician would do the same. The arrangement was conditional on both physicians adopting identical work modes used by Hadassah, and both would work under the supervision of Dr. Benno Gruenfelder, head of Hadassah's pediatrics department.

In May 1929, Dr. Yasski visited Haifa with Dr. Reuven Katzenelson, deputy director general of Hadassah. The two were surprised to find that despite the 1926 decision in favor of amalgamation of services, separate clinic hours were held for Hadassah infants and Kupat Holim infants and each of the physicians maintained his own statistical records. In a letter to Dr. Gruenfelder, Dr. Yasski and Dr. Katzenelson protested violation of the agreement:

> *To us, this arrangement appears abnormal. In our opinion, there should be no difference between Kupat Holim infants and other infants, and in the work of the Health Centers and in the field of modern medical work, it should be prohibited that such a division as this be made.*[350]

In the course of collaborative work, additional disagreements arose between Hadassah and Kupat Holim physicians, particularly surrounding feeding and nutrition of infants. Typical of the differences in approach, the physicians were divided regarding the appropriate time for giving children cod liver oil; Dr. Baruch Ostrowsky, a Hadassah physician, was in the habit of administering cod liver oil to healthy children from age three to four months, and even earlier to children with signs of rickets. On the other hand, Dr. Farber, a Kupat Holim physician, did not prescribe cod liver oil before the age of six months. Even the name "Health Center" lacked unanimous approval; Eliezer Perlson, the director general of Kupat Holim, even wrote Hadassah management in this regard, protesting: "We don't understand employment of such a broad name — 'health center' — when a more modest and suitable title could be used such as: 'care station for nursing babies.'" [351]

In order to settle disagreements and arrive at a unified approach to their work, Dr. Nissenboym suggested joint discussion among Hadassah and Kupat Holim physicians to reach a mutually acceptable position, but he stressed that "the opinion of Hadassah would be overriding."[352] The matter bothered Hadassah management. Dr. Yasski was disturbed that in most places Hadassah had succeeded in reaching a unified work mode except for Haifa, where, he claimed: "There are well-known conflicts and one must find the right way to work in cooperation."[353]

In July 1930, Dr. Yasski wrote the Kupat Holim executive in Tel Aviv to answer complaints that Hadassah was interfering in the work of Kupat Holim and entering into areas of activity that had been the prerogative of Kupat Holim. He argued:

> After all, Hadassah has 21 Health Centers around the country open to all social classes in the Yishuv, without payment. In the same places, Kupat Holim also operates its centers, yet we have never heard from Kupat Holim that we have entered a realm that doesn't belong to us.[354]

The two bodies — Hadassah and Kupat Holim — continued to work, each according to its own system, until 1935. Only then was a renewed attempt made to reach a unified approach. At a joint meeting between Hadassah, WIZO and Kupat Holim to formulate a joint organization for provision of public medicine in Haifa at all centers operated by the three organizations, it was decided that each center would provide services to residents in its own geographical area, without taking into account Kupat Holim membership. Additionally, a joint committee representing all centers would be formed with delegates from all three organizations, to decide on allocation of districts, contact and cooperation among centers and development of the network as a whole, to achieve collaboration. Also, Kupat Holim and WIZO would formulate a unified payment system in joint stations; Hadassah would not demand payment since it operated in distressed neighborhoods.[355]

In this manner the two health institutions achieved a unified and cooperative working relationship in the operation of Mother & Child Health Centers in Haifa.

We may assume that provision of health services was one of the areas where "control" of services constituted a "power base" within the Yishuv for opposing ideological positions within Zionism. Thus, in Tel Aviv there were tensions and power struggles over control of the first community hospital, Sha'ar Zion, that was rife with both personal and ideological rivalry. In Haifa — dubbed "Red Haifa"[356] due to the city's character as a socialist stronghold — difficulties in implementing agreements to amalgamate maternal and infant welfare services most probably reflected political undercurrents of antagonism between Hadassah and Socialist-oriented Kupat Holim — not just disagreements among professionals over childcare. Hadassah was an organization that, while officially apolitical, espoused a liberal "American" philosophy, which was at odds with the Socialists who at this time had a very different agenda. While there were attempts to "remove" maternal and infant welfare services as an arena for power politics, this was easier said than done — particularly in Red Haifa.

The Tiberias Health Center

Health Centers on the shore of the Sea of Galilee were established by a branch of the Hebrew Women's Federation that was established in Tiberias in January 1923 on the initiative of Bat-Sheva Kesselman, founder of the Jerusalem branch of the organization. The expressed purpose was "to aid indigent mothers in raising their children, reduce mortality among infants and cure children."[357] Tiberias was much in need of this kind of organization due to local conditions — a combination of a harsh climate, poverty, and poor hygiene and sanitation. Particularly during the hot summer months, disease (probably diarrhea) broke out, leading to a high incidence of infant mortality above the national average.

The response of the women of Tiberias was marked: Within five months of the founding of the branch, the Federation's Tiberias chapter had a hundred women volunteers in its ranks. The first Health Center was established in 1924. Managed at the beginning by Nurse Zelda Goldman, the Center had two units — a station for nursing babies and a *Tipat Chalav* station. The Center was unique in that from the outset it provided services for a mixed population of Jewish and Arab women at one facility.

The main difficulty facing the staff from the start was similar to those facing centers in Jerusalem and Haifa: initial lack of interest from mothers. Nurse Rachel Pesach described the situation as follows:

> As long as there was enough breast milk and the child developed, mothers saw no reason to come to the station. They did not understand the value of the work and its goal. Slowly [they] became accustomed to come with their infants and even stopped bringing sick children, becoming accustomed and understanding that the doctor's examination was not designed to cure, but to consult and guide [them] regarding maintenance and the nutritional status of their child.[358]

Over time, the nurses saw their systematic efforts bear fruit. They provided instruction for the mothers, and the mothers carefully followed their orders: to come to the Center only at appointed times; to nurse their children at regular intervals — they learned to go by the clock, which they had not used before; to prepare soups according to a nurse instructions; and to participate in courses for mothers run by the nurses. Monthly, Hadassah sent 80 kilograms of dry milk and 10 kilograms of buttermilk to the Center, at the organization's expense. The nurses provided diapers for a fee to mothers with large families who had no time to sew diapers for their babies, and even distributed cod liver oil. Over time, residents dubbed the Center the "School for Mothers" and the nurse was transformed into a popular local figure nicknamed "the Misses," leading to common usage such as "the Misses said... The Misses came... The Misses says to do such and such...."[359]

The fact that in May 1928 there was not one infant death in Tiberias was met with much jubilation, and Bertha Landsman praised the Center, writing: "The phenomenal absence of infant fatalities in Tiberias ... generated a sensation among the nurses. Tiberias was not included among the forty deaths we had [elsewhere] in May."[360]

Another unique characteristic of the Tiberias Center was adoption of "test feeding." When a mother had difficulty nursing her infant, the mother was brought to the Center for observation and guidance. According to this method, over a period of several days the mother arrived at the Center with her baby at 7 A.M. prior to the first feeding and left it at the Center for three to four hours until the second nursing, returning in this manner up until 5 P.M.

"Test feeding" had several objectives: The nurse taught the mother how to nurse and observed her while nursing; observation allowed the nurse to estimate the exact amount of milk the mother could provide her infant; the arrangement ensured the nurse that the mother had not fed her baby prior to bringing it to be weighed; and the system prevented spread of "feeding disorders" that led to hospitalization of infants.

Moreover, this system was adopted primarily among mothers who "were on such a low cultural level that the oral instructions they received from the nurse did not suffice at all."[361] Due to budgeting considerations, this system was not actualized in other centers, despite what was viewed as "splendid results."

For the mothers' comfort, Landsman ordered special chairs for nursing mothers. She described their design as "...according to the regular proportions of a chair for an adult but an unusual leg height suited to the requirements of a nursing mother, without needing to use a footstool for her legs during nursing."[362]

The Safed Health Center

In February 1923, a branch of the Hebrew Women's Federation was established in Safed, a town in the hills of the Central Galilee. The organization attracted some 50 members during the first five months of operation. Among social welfare activities on the agenda, the members planned to establish a *Tipat Chalav* station, but lack of funding prevented actualization of this plan.

In Safed, assistance to pregnant women, women after childbirth and their infants was carried out on an individual basis by caretakers in the homes of the recipients. During the first year of activity, the Hebrew Women's Federation assisted the caretakers by bringing a midwife to Safed and paying her salary; attending to supply of diapers and underclothes for newborns; providing money for new mothers to buy foodstuffs; supplying milk to mothers who could not nurse; and calling in a midwife at the designated time. The caretaker assisted the expectant woman from the first month of pregnancy due to fear of miscarriage, and in such cases called in a doctor. From the seventh month of gestation, the caretaker ensured the woman would be under medical supervision, and assisted in preparation of equipment needed during childbirth. During the first week after delivery, she stayed in the home of the new mother to tend to housekeeping duties and buy food for the family, while supervising the health of mother and child. Supervision of mother and child continued for three to four weeks. If living conditions in the home were very poor — if the mother did not have a bed and delivery at home was inappropriate — the caretaker arranged for a hospital delivery.

The need for a Health Center in Safed grew greater; the chairperson of the local branch of the Hebrew Women's Federation underscored the situation, stressing: "The city sits in a remote location and the Jews have almost no source of livelihood, and there are many poor, particularly among the Sephardic Jews."[363]

In December 1923 the Hebrew Women's Federation turned to Szold to request aid in establishing a *Tipat Chalav* station and a station for care of nursing babies.

Szold appreciated their initiatives and endeavors, but was unable to assist, except for two small donations received at her office that she decided to grant to Safed. The first — a $25 donation from the Montefiore Women's Federation in Atlantic City, New Jersey — was accompanied by a note of encouragement and praise of their work: "It is clear to me that to maintain a Federation of this kind in a remote place like Safed requires an extraordinary effort of perseverance and steadfastness."[364]

The second donation — 2.18 Eretz Israel pounds — was earmarked to help support provision of milk in special cases: "...to supply milk to nursing mothers that do not have the ability to pay to obtain milk, and particularly supply milk to poor nursing babies in need of such."[365]

Only in November 1929 did the Hebrew Women's Federation in Safed succeed in opening a Health Center. Backing, however, was only sufficient for six months' rent of the facility chosen to house the Center. Nevertheless, the Center was opened despite apprehension concerning the future in light of lack of additional funding from Hadassah or the Hebrew Women's Federation. Hadassah paid the salary of the nurse but was unable to provide more than that, warning: "The Women's Federation must know that if other sources for this objective are not found, the Center will be closed."[366] The attending physician, Dr. P. Vail, aware of the importance of the Center for Safed residents, suggested that residents participate in maintaining the facility. The proposal was adopted.

The Center, which included operation of the nursing babies' station, operated on the Sabbath. However, Landsman objected to this arrangement, demanding closure of the station on the Sabbath, asserting that Hadassah upheld the principle of six workdays a week, eight hours a day. The weekly day of rest for the nurses was Saturday, therefore the Center should not be open on Saturdays "except in cases of calamity under special circumstances."[367]

Landsman opposed breaking religious laws "when it is not necessary. It is presumptuous to work [on the Sabbath] among residents of Safed." She knew that Safed, for centuries a center of Jewish mysticism, was characterized by a deeply religious Jewish community and therefore operation on the Sabbath was deemed particularly inappropriate.

According to the reports of Nurse Chedva Hilper regarding operation of the station for nursing babies, on a monthly basis from November 1931 to October 1933, the Center in Safed provided services to an average of 15 pregnant women, 30 babies up to the age of 12 months, and 45 infants above the age of one year. She noted that those mothers who visited the Center on a regular basis were mostly of Ashkenazi origin, while few Sephardic mothers sought the Center's services.

There were two underlying reasons for scanty attendance: First of all, harsh economic situations prompted many families to leave Safed and the number of pregnant women dropped. Moreover, among those who remained, difficulties tied to unemployment and the struggle to make a living — a war of survival — demanded most of the attention and energy of residents. Secondly, during the 1929 Arab riots[368] the Hebrew Women's Federation provided material assistance to needy families; however, with the end of violence, assistance was discontinued and the mothers stopped coming to the Center.

On the other hand, Hilper noted that overall, the health status of babies cared for at the Center was "very good," underscoring this fact by noting that the percentage of infant mortality was negligible and "cases of death were almost non-existent."[369]

The nurses conducted lectures on nutrition and cleanliness and taught mothers how to protect their children from diseases. Compliance of mothers was incomplete, but some of them strictly followed the instructions regarding hygiene: They learned to bathe their children regularly despite the shortage of water, took their children out in the open air even in cold weather, and learned to take care of proper nutrition of their children. She summed up the situation by concluding that "all in all, everything is fine from a developmental standpoint."[370] There was one problem, however, that the nurses were unable to overcome — the problem of the kind of milk mothers were in the habit of giving their children: goat's milk, deemed "highly undesirable" by the nurses. She noted that economics played a decisive role: "We have been unable to beat this stumbling block, for this milk is cheaper [than cow's milk]."[371]

Health Centers in Tel Aviv

In Tel Aviv, maternal and child welfare was dealt with by two women's organizations: Hadassah and WIZO (Women's International Zionist Organization). While in other cities in Eretz Israel, Hadassah and the Hebrew Women's Federation maintained a cooperative relationship, in Tel Aviv a working relationship often failed to materialize.

WIZO began operating in Eretz Israel in 1920, following a decision made at the founding convention of WIZO in London to open a central office in Eretz Israel. The first activities of the organization were in Tel Aviv and Jaffa, initiated by a number of volunteers. At the time, there was already an active branch of the Hebrew Women's Federation in Jerusalem and the first buds of a branch in Haifa. The volunteers, all local women, guided mothers — primarily new immigrants — in raising their children. Only in 1927 did the women organize within a broader framework called the National Federation, a body subordinate to WIZO headquarters in London. The organization found itself in conflict with two other women's organizations: the local organization, the Hebrew Women's Federation, which saw the new body as a rival for resources in funding and membership, and with Hadassah, the American organization that viewed with disfavor ties between women's frameworks in Eretz Israel and other organizations abroad, particularly those in Europe. Nevertheless, over the years the organizations cooperated, and in 1933 it was decided to establish one united Zionist Women's Federation in Eretz Israel — a joint framework amalgamating WIZO nationwide and the Hebrew Women's Federation.[372]

WIZO's and Hadassah's first volunteer work began in 1924, providing for the welfare of new mothers. WIZO from New Zealand opened a station to care for pregnant women in the Neve Shalom neighborhood of Tel Aviv. For this purpose WIZO underwrote the cost of sending two nurses to England to study the Plunkett System — a special method of caring for new mothers and infants popular in England, New Zealand and Australia at the time. Dr. Theodore Zlocisti, who was responsible for supervising the nursing station established by the Tel Aviv branch of WIZO, was appointed director of the Neve Shalom station.

Hadassah, struggling with financial problems of its own, had not yet established a Health Center in Tel Aviv. It did, however, send a midwife from Jerusalem to Jaffa to assist women who delivered their babies in their homes. A join committee with the *Ezer Yoldot* (Assistance to New Mother's) Society and the Hebrew Women's Federation paid the midwife's salary of 10 Eretz Israel pounds a month and assisted impoverished new mothers. Parental and gynecological work was carried out in Dr. Yosef Asherman's clinic in Tel Aviv, while two Hadassah nurses conducted home visits and advised pregnant women registered at his clinic.

Two of the first Hadassah Health Centers in Tel Aviv were established with the assistance of the Nathan Straus Fund. The Fund even supported the facilities during their first year of operation. The two centers were opened on November 1, 1926 — one in the Neve Shaanan neighborhood, the other in the Geulah neighborhood on Yona Hanavi Street. The two centers operated according to a collaborative arrangement reached between Kupat Holim and Hadassah. The agreement stipulated:

Hadassah operated the centers for nursing babies, appointed the medical personnel and covered their maintenance.

Visiting hours for mothers and babies were carried out on separate days for Hadassah and members of Kupat Holim.

Kupat Holim opened a milk kitchen in one of the two centers. The milk was prepared according to the directives of a Kupat Holim physician for nursing babies registered with Kupat Holim. With the approval of a Kupat Holim physician, milk was also supplied — for a fee — to infants whose parents were not Kupat Holim members.

Hadassah appointed kitchen personnel and provided equipment for pasteurization.

The Health Centers were named after Kupat Holim and Hadassah.[373]

On December 5, 1926, a third Health Center was inaugurated on Nechemia Street, to care for infants in the Yemenite Quarter of Tel Aviv. The Center was launched by WIZO. The new Center provided services for children up to the age of two; older children were referred to one of the two other centers run by Hadassah.

The procedures at WIZO Health Centers were different from those of Hadassah, a source of harsh clashes between the management of the two organizations. WIZO Centers were run according to the Plunkett System, which was based on three principles: supportive "propaganda" in favor of breast feeding the infant; enriching the child's diet with cream; and massaging the breasts to generate a richer milk supply.[374]

Hadassah management and its physicians, particularly Dr. Gruenfelder — the pediatrician responsible for overseeing the work of Hadassah Health Centers — was opposed to this method, claiming it was not suitable for the climate and character of Eretz Israel. Most of the mothers were not in need of "supportive propaganda"; 98% of the children were breast-fed. The only "propaganda" mothers needed was encouragement to limit the number of feedings and length of feedings per day. (Moreover, most of the women from Oriental backgrounds continued to nurse for over a year.) The second principle was also unsuitable, for during the long summer months — April through October — infants should not be given food rich in fat. As for the third principle, Hadassah physicians also assigned importance to massaging, in cases where it was necessary. However, they objected strongly to nurses dealing with this issue, arguing this was an invasion into the medical realm — the province of physicians only.[375]

Organization of Work

The WIZO Health Center offered advice and instruction regarding infants only up to the age of two. In other words, children over the age of two were left without any hygienic supervision, or were transferred to Hadassah Health Centers. Pregnant women received care and guidance only at Hadassah Health Centers. Hadassah management objected to this, claiming that treatment was fragmented. Dr. Yasski argued: "Care of the pregnant woman is an integral part of care of the infant."[376] Consequently, Hadassah management demanded that the WIZO Center change its format and provide health care for the entire family — pregnant women, infants and toddlers (age two to four) — as in Hadassah Health Centers.

Nursing Staff

The nurses working in Hadassah Health Centers were graduates of Hadassah's nursing school. There were also registered nurses who had undergone further training in public nursing, whose base income was 9 Eretz Israel pounds a month. Nurses in WIZO Health Centers were caretakers (*metaplot*) for infants and toddlers and had studied at WIZO's school for training caretakers, whose basic income was 7.5 Eretz Israel pounds a month. Only the head nurse at WIZO facilities was a registered nurse. The two nurses who had been sent to England for special training taught the caretakers the Plunkett System.

Aware of the gap in these different work methods, Hadassah management argued that lack of a unified approach between Hadassah and WIZO led to waste and inefficiency in utilization of human resources and put a strain on most families by requiring unnecessary visits. For instance, an infant registered at the WIZO nursing babies station received home visits from a WIZO nurse, while its older sibling, under the supervision of Hadassah, received home visits from a Hadassah nurse — clearly, this task could be covered by one qualified nurse in a single visit. Hadassah held that this state of affairs could not be allowed to continue and a way must be found to cooperate and unify operations and eliminate redundancies. Hadassah held that the WIZO station must adopt Hadassah's setup.

To create an organizational tie and find ways to arrive at a common approach, the two federations engaged in drawn-out negotiations. As a first step, a committee was organized, comprised of delegates from the Tel Aviv Municipality and nurses from both Hadassah and WIZO frameworks. Many of the committee's meetings were devoted to formulating mutually acceptable care procedures and reorganizing public health services in Tel Aviv. In the end, it was decided to appoint a preparatory committee to work out a unification scheme. The committee included two delegates from Hadassah, Professor Israel Kligler and Dr. Benno Gruenfelder; two delegates from WIZO, Dr. Theodore Zlocisti and Hadassah Samuel, chairperson of WIZO in Eretz Israel; and two delegates from the Tel Aviv Municipality, H. Gelner, director of the Childcare Department, and Shoshana Persitz, head of the Education Department.[377]

The preparatory committee made the following decisions: WIZO would expand its operation of Health Centers and add advice and instruction for "children in passage" (ages three to four) and pregnant women; a common budget would be drawn up for all Health Centers in Tel Aviv, and four bodies would share expenditures: Hadassah, WIZO, the Tel Aviv Municipality, and the parents.

Persitz was the first to introduce a system of nominal fees for services rendered to mothers in Health Centers. She argued in favor of "a grush [a coin of nominal value] per mother per month." Payment was based on investigation of the welfare status of the family. Mothers without means received services gratis.

In regard to a program for unifying care of children and pregnant women, delegates from the three bodies all agreed to adopt care procedures used by Hadassah. That is to say:

- Supervision of hygiene encompassing the entire family: pregnant women, infants and children up to the age of four
- A unified system of managing Health Centers
- Equal pay and identical uniforms for nurses
- A uniform method of daily and monthly record keeping by each nurse and each Center
- Joint management[378]

To carry out the plan in practice, Tel Aviv — then a city of 50,000 inhabitants — was divided into four regions, each with its own regional Health Center: Health Center A run by Hadassah in the northern sector, and Health Centers B, C and D run by WIZO in the center and southern sectors of the city.

Each center encompassed the following scope of care: Pregnant women received monthly examination and nutrition guidance. During the first year of life, infants (children between the ages of 10 days and 12 months) were to visit the center weekly and a physician would examine each child during reception hours; toddlers (children between the ages of one and four years)[379] were to visit the center once every two weeks, and the physician would examine each child three times a year. "Children in passage," between the end of the third year and the end of the fourth year, were to visit the center once every two months and would be examined by the doctor once a year. At the end of the fourth year, the doctor was to conduct a final checkup, at which time the center would grant a transfer document to kindergarten. Kindergarteners, between the ages four and six, were to be examined twice a year by a physician. For schoolchildren, medical examination and health education would be carried out at school by the nurse and doctor.

According to the new arrangement, the following working principles were adopted: Concentration of children and pregnant women in a geographical area would ensure uniform, systematic, comprehensive care with follow-up from the day of birth to the end of school. Each center would enjoy managerial independence; administration would be placed in the hands of the physician or chief nurse. A Hadassah nurse-supervisor would oversee work of the nurses in all centers. Home visits would be carried out by one nurse per family. Centers would not provide care for sick children. A uniform fee would be levied on mothers by the municipal social welfare department according to the situation of the family. A governing committee composed of delegates of the three bodies — Dr. Yasski for Hadassah, Dr. Zlocisti for WIZO and Y. Rokach from the Tel Aviv Municipality — would coordinate work between the centers.

Toward the end of 1934, Hadassah management began to plan the transfer of its Health Centers to the responsibility of the Tel Aviv Municipality, transforming them into municipal facilities in every way. Collaboration between Hadassah and WIZO encountered many difficulties. WIZO wished to free itself entirely from responsibility for the joint centers and to devote itself only to its own Mother & Child Care Centers, which mainly provided intensive nurturing and convalescence for infants in need of special care. Thus, there was no alternative but to transfer the responsibility for WIZO centers to the Tel Aviv Municipality and Hadassah.

Kupat Holim demanded that it be a participant in the governing committee — however, Dr. Yasski made this conditional on Kupat Holim assuming financial and administrative responsibility for a number of Health Centers. Dr. Yosef Meir, who conducted negotiations in the name of the Kupat Holim, replied to Dr. Yasski that the Kupat Holim did not have the budget for this, but could help by providing medical services and collecting payment. Moreover, if its demand to join the governing committee was not met, Dr. Meir declared that Kupat Holim would establish its own Heath Centers for its members, as it had done in Haifa. Dr. Yasski opposed what he labeled "the isolationist tendencies of Kupat

Holim"[380] but expressed hopes that Kupat Holim would at least carry out "complete and not partial work"[381] in its centers — that is, encompass hygiene supervision for the entire family from the pregnant woman to children in kindergarten, including home visits. At a meeting held in December 1934, Kupat Holim agreed to take financial and administrative responsibilities for the Health Center in North Tel Aviv, and a Kupat Holim delegate was added to the governing committee.[382]

In 1935, Kupat Holim opened a Health Center on Ben-Zion Street in Tel Aviv. The Center was designed to serve both Kupat Holim members and the general public. In the same year, WIZO curtailed its own operation, and its delegate withdrew from the governing committee.[383] In June 1935, WIZO closed its Health Center on Carmel Street and ceased providing care for pregnant women at its two remaining centers in the Yemenite Quarter and the Neve Shalom neighborhood. As a result, women were left without a Health Center; the governing committee was convened to deal with the crisis and formulate a program to distribute the women among Hadassah and Kupat Holim centers. It was decided that each center would treat pregnant women and infants whether they were members of Kupat Holim or not, and all centers would be under the supervision of the governing committee. On the July 17, 1935, a fifth regional Health Center was opened in the center of the city, in the Straus Health House — most of the children who had been registered at the Carmel Street Center were transferred there. In August 1935, a sixth regional Health Center was inaugurated on Neve Shaanan Street.[384]

In April 1936, a move was launched to transfer all the stations for nursing babies to municipal auspices.[385] Dr. Abraham Katzenelson, director of the Health Department of the National Committee, was opposed to what he perceived as "dismantling the preventive project that more than any other medical project demands a uniform method, concentrated professional supervision and unified management."[386]

Dr. Katzenelson suggested that Hadassah continue to administer the project and remain responsible for operations — with the aid of the governing committee that would be composed of delegates from Hadassah and the Tel Aviv Municipality. In the meantime, the Tel Aviv Municipality would be asked "to refrain from any action that might disintegrate the public medicine project."[387] Due to some of the personnel opposition, transfer of authority was delayed; however, finally, on the August 1, 1936, Hadassah Health Centers were transferred to the responsibility and administration of the Tel Aviv Municipality.[388]

Summary

Description of the process that led to the establishment of the first Health Centers in Eretz Israel and their work in the field of health and education of young mothers and children, including details of the difficulties encountered in their establishment and operation, underscore the centers' pioneering but decisive role in providing guidance and instruction to pregnant women and mothers in the care of their children. The success of these endeavors, which evolved into a nationwide program carried out in keeping with a uniform format initially developed by Hadassah, required a large degree of good will and cooperation between three complementary but at times competing organizations with similar aims: Hadassah, WIZO and Kupat Holim.

Hadassah's ultimate goal was to lay the foundations and create the infrastructure for a public health system based on a unified and comprehensive line of action organized as a national network that could eventually be transferred to the responsibility of the Yishuv itself. From a historic viewpoint, the Health Centers championed by Hadassah were created from scratch, ushering in a new era regarding preventive medical care for expectant women, mothers and children in Eretz Israel.

It is important to note that from the beginning of its activities in Eretz Israel, Hadassah planned to transfer all its services to the authority of the Yishuv when the local community would be strong enough to maintain its medical needs on its own. In 1931, the Hadassah hospital in Tel Aviv was transferred to municipal authority and the Hadassah hospital in Haifa was turned over to the local Jewish community. The two hospitals were promised initial financial backing to be phased out gradually over five years. In 1930, Hadassah organized the *Kupat Holim Amamit* (Popular Sick Fund), transferring medical services in rural settlements to its authority, while providing annual backing. Responsibility for the hospital in Tiberias was also transferred to the Yishuv, and Hadassah continued to provide the annual budget. In 1936, proactive medical services such as the Mother & Child Health Centers, were scheduled to be transferred to the National Committee, the self-governing body of the Yishuv — however, the outbreak of the 1936–1939 Arab Revolt forced a delay, as the community was unable to assume the heavy financial burden at that juncture. In the meantime, Hadassah expanded its proactive activities, in keeping with the most urgent needs of the growing Yishuv. Only proactive medical services in Tel Aviv were transferred to the Municipality at the end of the summer 1935.

E. The Educational-Health Program

Hadassah management understood from the outset of its operation in Eretz Israel that preventive medicine could not be limited only to a portion of the population that was in need of massive assistance and guidance. It must encompass the entire public — rich and poor. The preferred system that ought to be adopted was education of mothers — all mothers. Health Centers served as a central tool in realizing this goal.

Educational-health work began with care of the expectant mother from the beginning of her pregnancy. It then expanded, encompassing delivery of her offspring and postnatal care extending through age two to four years, and concluding with care of the kindergartener (age four to six years). Upon entering elementary school, the schoolchild became the responsibility of a separate agency — the School Hygiene Department.

The goals of educational-health work were defined as follows:

Teach and instill basic rules of hygiene; support, aid and instruct expectant women during pregnancy; teach and guide mothers in infant nutrition; encourage and extend breast feeding; guide mothers in the transfer from breast milk to milk substitutes; care for supply of pasteurized milk and teach proper preparation of food by the mother in the home; educate, advise and instruct mothers in the raising of their children; teach mothers how to prevent disease stemming from improper nutrition or lack of hygiene; conduct home visits to locate all families in need and provide support; advance the health of each child in the family; locate and address defects in need of rectification; and improve Health Centers and encourage mothers to use their services.

Organization of Work

Care for expectant women was not only designed to ensure a healthy and normal pregnancy without complications and to provide postnatal supervision to maintain the health of the mother. It was assumed that an ongoing relationship with the doctor and nurses at the center would build a foundation for guiding the mother in the care of her future offspring. Therefore, the work program was divided into five areas of activity, realized through close cooperation between Hadassah and the Hebrew Women's Federation: care of expectant women; assistance to new mothers; care of nursing infants; distribution of milk through *Tipat Chalav*; and care of "children in passage" between the ages of two and four.

Care of Expectant Women

Care of expectant women was divided into three periods: during gestation, during childbirth, and post-delivery.

Registration: Expectant women registered at the Health Center closest to their home, no later than the fourth month of pregnancy. At first it was necessary to locate the women and convince them to register at Health Centers; however, over time women began to come on their own.

Visits to Health Centers: During the first two trimesters, expectant women were examined once a week; during the seventh and eighth month of gestation, once every two weeks; and in the ninth month, every week.

Routine Lab Work: On the first visit to the center, blood and urine samples were taken and tested, including blood sugar levels. Protein levels in urine were monitored and weight gain recorded during every subsequent visit. Blood pressure was routinely checked by the nurse. Women in need of dental care were referred to a dentist; needy women received free dental care.

Instruction: Each woman received individualized guidance during her visit to the Health Center regarding hygiene during pregnancy, preparation of clothing for her infant and herself, and immediate care of the newborn.

Center nurses also conducted group instruction for expectant women under the guidance of Dr. Gruenfelder, the gynecologists working at the Health Center, and the head nurse Bertha Landsman. Subject matter included aspects of pregnancy and birth such as preparation for delivery of their infants, development of the fetus and care of the newborn. The nurse explained female physiology — the structure of the reproductive organs, conception, the role of the placenta, and development of the fetus in the womb. Women were instructed in nutrition, including proper diet during pregnancy — explanations were given about basic food elements, the functions of each, and what foods were recommended and not recommended during pregnancy — while striving to instill the rule of thumb that a pregnant women "did not have to eat for two, but rather eat the right food."[389] Participants learned proper hygiene and body cleanliness during pregnancy, including instruction to wash their nipples daily with water and alcohol, and the importance of breast-feeding because mother's milk had all the elements needed for building the body of the infant.[390]

The nurses were instructed how to arrange their presentation. They were told to prepare seating for all mothers. Proper demeanor was stressed: "[Nurses should] speak very slowly in vocabulary suitable for understanding, so the women will absorb the content of the discussion."[391]

It was suggested that they should explain and demonstrate their points using models and pictures. Moreover, nurses were instructed to check every subject before making recommendations to mothers. Thus, in regard to nutrition, the price of fruits and vegetables in the local market should be checked before recommending buying them.

House Visits: During the seventh month of pregnancy, the nurse conducted a house visit to evaluate socio-economic conditions in the home and prepare the women for labor. A second visit was conducted after delivery, to evaluate the health status of the mother and to give her practical advice about care for her newborn. Home visits served not only as an integral part of supervision and instruction, but also as a way to gain the trust of the family, as Bertha Landsman said: "Only on this condition does the success of the work of public nurses hinge."[392]

Assistance to New Mothers

Expectant women were instructed to complete all preparations for childbirth six weeks before term. The women already knew whether they were supposed to go to the maternity ward in the hospital or whether a midwife would assist them in their homes. If it was to be a home delivery, the mother was instructed to prepare the room where she would go into labor — clean the room, remove all upholstered furniture and rugs and prepare necessary equipment: bandages, Lysol, alcohol, talcum powder, boric acid and a hefty quantity of bed linen and clothing for the newborn. The women were enjoined: "Take the advice of the doctor, not your neighbor, and don't wait for the last minute."[393]

After childbirth: New mothers were instructed to stay in bed at least a week and to refrain from all strenuous tasks for a month. The rationale given the women: "So your milk will not spoil, and your baby suffer the consequences."[394]

The Hebrew Women's Federation sent a volunteer to visit each new mother to help keep house during the first week of recuperation after delivery. Needy mothers received funding for milk, sugar, meat and poultry. (In Jerusalem, for example, each needy mother received half a kilogram each of sugar, tea, cocoa, meat and poultry, and two liters of milk — according to the doctor's recommendation.)

Home Visits: The nurse conducted a home visit to instruct the new mother in matters of hygiene and nursing, demonstrating how to bathe the baby and how to fulfill the infant's needs, making sure the mother understood her instructions and the doctor's orders — and carried them out in practice.

Care of Nursing Babies

Instruction for mothers was conducted at two junctures when the nurse's skills as an instructional nurse were called into service. The first was individual instruction in the home of the new mother during the nurse's post-delivery home visit and when the new mother brought her infant to the Health Center for advice. The second was group instruction for mothers at the Health Center. Guidance was given in a series of meetings, and discussions geared to prepare the future mother for her role.

The course curriculum covered the following subjects:

The room and infant's cradle: Mothers were instructed to prepare a crib or cradle or large basket for the baby and not to leave it in the mother's bed, warning the women: "You might harm or suffocate it during your sleep."

The women were told to spread a net over the baby's bed to keep away flies and misquotes that would disrupt sleep and could carry disease.

Sleep: The women were instructed to accustom their babies to sleeping at regular intervals. The infant should sleep at least six hours straight during the night, taking a long nap after breakfast and a short nap in the afternoon. The mother was instructed not to let her infant sleep in the late afternoon hours, so it would not be up all night. While the child was sleeping, the room should be well ventilated, dimly lit and quiet. The position of the infant should be shifted from time to time. Mothers were admonished: "Don't keep [the infant] awake in the evenings to amuse the family — a child is not a toy."

Clothing: Baby apparel should be simple, soft and easy to launder. The infant's wardrobe should contain gowns, socks and diapers. Clothing should vary from summer to winter. The baby's head should not be covered when the child was in the house. Clothes should be changed morning and evening. Diapers should be changed whenever they were wet. In a number of Health Centers sewing circles were organized where women gathered to receive instruction in sewing baby clothes from a Hebrew Women's Federation volunteer who was an experienced seamstress.

Bathing: Mothers should accustom their newborn from birth to being bathed at regular intervals — either before the second morning feeding or before going to sleep at night. Water should be tepid. A clean towel and clean clothes should be at hand and talcum should be used to powder sensitive areas. The baby's eyes and mouth should be washed twice a day with cool boiled water and the child should be examined to ensure there were no skin blemishes on the child's scalp.

Nutrition: Mothers were instructed to nurse their babies themselves. The reason given: "Children fed mother's milk are generally more robust children."

Breast milk was the best nourishment, but if it was given in a careless and disorderly manner, it could be detrimental, they were told. The infant should be fed regularly every three hours by the clock. Even if the infant was sleeping, it should be awakened at regular intervals to be nursed. Nursing should last five to twenty minutes, according to the needs of the child and the quantity of milk the mother had. The baby should be given cool boiled water to drink a number of times a day. The mother was instructed to take care of her health "...so her milk will be beneficial to her nursing infant."

If there was not enough breast milk, the mother should supplement with cow's milk, or wean the child and feed it only cow's milk (whole milk, milk diluted in water, milk with sugar or other elements) as directed by the physician, and of course "only if the doctor ordered the child be given [other] milk." At six months, upon doctor's orders, the child received a small portion of well-cooked lentils once a day and was gradually weaned by the end of the first year of life. If the mother continued to nurse beyond a year, she was told: "The only outcome is that the mother is weakened, without benefit to the child."

Mothers were instructed to adhere to a rigid feeding schedule and not to feed their child at night, even if it cried. Indeed, mothers became accustomed to regular feedings and there were those who told the nurses that they had clocks repaired that had not been in use in their houses for ages, in order to take care to nurse at set intervals.

Health

Regular visits and checkups at the Health Centers were graduated, according to the needs of the child.

During every visit during the first five months, infants were weighed, and then again at age six months and a year. Height and head measurements were taken four times during the first year of life. The child's *fonticulus*, the soft spot on its skull, was measured by a physician when the child reached the age of 12 months.

The first home visit was conducted after delivery. The second visit was carried out when the child's diet was changed to solid food. Other visits were scheduled if and when need arose. When a mother did not visit the center even after she was summoned, a nurse was sent to the home.

Each baby was vaccinated against smallpox and diphtheria. Additional vaccinations were administered as needed, according to directives from the Mandatory government's Health Department.

During visits, mothers were instructed to take their children out in the open air twice daily, while avoiding dusty environments, drafts and places where sunrays fell directly on the infant's face. They were told not to hold their babies more than necessary. If the infant developed diarrhea and threw up, they were to feed it cool water only and call the doctor immediately. If the baby cried, the mother should investigate the reason and not try to solve the problem by immediate feeding. If the baby did not cease crying, a doctor should be called. Mothers were told they were responsible for an atmosphere conducive to their child's well being — laundering its diapers, airing out the cradle, and maintaining a regular daily schedule of three hours between feedings. The nurses underscored these directives, stressing "...order and cleanliness are the infant's best friend."

Nurses at Health Centers recommended the following daily regime:

6:00 A.M.	First morning feeding
6:00–8:00 A.M.	Play in the cradle
8:30 A.M.	Bath
9:00 A.M.	Second morning feeding
9:00–Noon	Long nap (with open windows)
Noon	Noon feeding
3:00–5:00 P.M.	Afternoon stroll — weather permitting
5:00 P.M.	Change of clothes or bath
6:00 P.M.	Evening feeding before bed
10:00 P.M.	Nighttime feeding

The nurses used all kinds of incentives to attract the mothers to the Health Centers to receive instruction and "convince" them to follow their recommendations. One of the incentives was "prizes" for "outstanding mothers" who came regularly to the Health Center and strictly followed nurses' directives. The prizes were distributed at a well-attended neighborhood celebration held once a year at the Health Center. Two months prior to the event, the nurse began "propagandizing" among mothers who visited the center, announcing that *"Tipat Chalav* plans to give prizes to mothers who care for their children well, according to directives."[395] The upcoming event was publicized throughout the neighborhood and in local papers "to encourage mothers to make efforts to care for their babies."[396]

At the beginning, there were mothers who did not comprehend the meaning of the celebration. In one report it was noted:

> *[Some thought] that prizes were being given for the most beautiful or largest infant. When they understood the purpose, the mothers began to flood the center to ask the staff questions about everything not clear to them about care of babies, being most curious to know what the prizes were...until it was explained that the best prize was the health of their infant — in that the mother was fulfilling everything according to directives.*[397]

The celebration was held in the courtyard of the Health Center which was decorated with flags and banners emblazoned with the Hadassah motto *Arucat bat ami* (Healing of my People) and various catch phrases, including "The world does not exist except for the utterances of infants" (a play on words of a popular adage) and "The most splendid sights on earth are stars, flowers and a child's two eyes."[398]

The event was attended by mothers from the neighborhood with their children — including those who had never visited the Health Center — together with honored guests, including delegates from the Hebrew Women's Federation, Kupat Holim, Hadassah personnel, and the neighborhood governing committee (i.e., a kind of semi-official residents' organization).

The ceremony followed a fixed pattern: The nurses reviewed the work of the Health Center and the doctor described developments, stressing the importance of the center's work in reducing infant mortality. The highpoint of the celebration was the allocation of prizes to outstanding mothers. Excellence was based on three basic criteria: 1. excellence in general concern for the infant; 2. expression of faith and trust in the center's physician and nurses; 3. regular attendance at the center and fulfillment of directives.

Several examples regarding the identity of the recipients serve to illustrate what constituted "excellence" in the eyes of the organizers. One Outstanding Mother from Haifa had given birth to a baby weighing 1,800 grams. The mother had a heart and lung condition and physicians had forbidden her to nurse her infant. Nevertheless, she had partially nursed the newborn until it was weaned to a milk substitute. At the time of the celebration, the baby was eight months old and reported to be "entirely healthy and of good weight."[399] The prize: two sheets, two towels, two pillows and two dressing gowns. In Jerusalem, according to reports, the prize had been awarded to an Ashkenazi man whose wife had given birth to a male child. The mother fell ill and remained hospitalized for an extended period. The father visited the Health Center regularly with his newborn son, learning to prepare a formula, to cook cereals and vegetable soup. It was noted that the father closely followed the directives he received from the nurses, stressing: "[He] acted toward them with all the seriousness and trust required and succeeded by this devotion in bringing up [the infant] under good and normal circumstances, and was rewarded by the satisfaction of seeing him prosper."[400] The prize: a sweater and hat for the baby.

In Safed a single prize was given to a mother "for excellence in devoted and rational care of her daughter."[401] The prize: the Education Department exempted the Outstanding Mother from payment of tuition during the 1933–1934 school year for one of her children enrolled in a school run by the Department.

At the end of the event, it was tradition for a number of mothers to thank the medical staff. At a celebration in Tiberias, three mothers were chosen to fulfill this task: two Jewish mothers, one of Ashkenazi origin and one of Sephardic origin, and a Christian mother. The Ashkenazi mother thanked the staff for their care during her pregnancy, for providing a midwife and for teaching her how to feed her infant. The Sephardic mother related how all her fears and worries about her infant disappeared immediately upon visiting the Health Center. The Arab Christian mother thanked the nurses for teaching her how to feed and care for her children. The mothers all emphasized the assistance and guidance they received from doctors and nurses.[402]

There were mothers who felt insulted that they did not receive a prize although they followed directives and their babies were healthy. It was explained to them that "their care was on behalf of their babies and not in order to receive a prize"[403] and they were ensured that celebrations were held from time to time, and in the future they would be able "to show the public the results of their infallible care."[404]

Milk Distribution

Hadassah management became convinced that there was no value in allocation of milk without integrating it with the care of nursing babies. Therefore, directives were issued not to distribute milk to every mother who requested it. Milk was allocated only to new mothers in need, for a nominal fee — and only with the approval of a physician. Mothers of means paid the full cost of the milk, while needy mothers paid according to their abilities. Milk was supplied by dairy farms under hygienic supervision and was required to contain a set percentage of fat. The milk was pasteurized, mixed with water and sugar according to doctor's orders, and poured into bottles with special caps, then sterilized. In the summer, milk was kept on ice.

Hadassah's milk distribution program deviated from the organization's policy of engaging in preventive medicine that focused on educational-medical activities. Yet, the positive effect of providing *limited* material assistance through the distribution of milk to babies from needy families registered at the Health Centers. An activity carried out in collaboration with charitable organizations was a positive instrument in achieving Hadassah's primary role and goals: enhancing preventive medicine.

From reports written by the Health Centers in Eretz Israel — drawn from reports from five stations for nursing babies operating in Jerusalem in 1929 and reflected in the table below — it becomes apparent that guidance provided at the centers and the distribution of pasteurized milk significantly contributed to the reduction in infant mortality.

Reduction in Mortality Among Five Jerusalem Stations[405]

Year	1931	1932	1933	1934
# of children registered at the station	3582	4057	4488	4513
# of children who died	173	153	167	133
Percent of deaths	4.8%	3.8%	3.7%	2.9%

Cooperation in Tipat Chalav between Hadassah and the Hebrew Women's Federation

Distribution of milk was carried out with close collaboration between Hadassah and the Hebrew Women's Federation, through a special budget provided by Hadassah women in America, funded from donations and what was labeled the *Tipat Chalav* Fund.[406] Hadassah was responsible for supervision of hygiene at the farm and dairy that supplied milk to *Tipat Chalav*, in particular to ensure the cows were clean and healthy.[407] Milk samples were taken daily to guarantee milk was clean and met quality standards. Hadassah sent an experienced nurse to each city to organize *Tipat Chalav* stations, paying for the milk, rent, a janitor, furnishings and equipment including bottles and suitable caps, sugar, groats, ice and so forth.

"Children-in-Passage"

At age two, toddlers registered at the station for nursing babies were transferred to the care of the Children-in-Passage Department (ages three to four) where the growing child was monitored up to the age of four. The nurses were told not to allow mothers to abandon the Health Center when their children turned four, but rather to encourage them to continue to come at appointed times so nurses could follow their growth. The nurses were instructed specifically by Bertha Landsman, chief nurse of Hadassah, "...to make all possible endeavors to keep under the supervision of the center as much as possible as many babies in the ages 3–4 from outside — even if they had not attended the center previously."[408]

Landsman compared the data from the records of all Health Centers in Eretz Israel regarding children-in-passage. She found that in 1931, in the five Jerusalem centers, there were 1,038 children of this age registered, while in Haifa there were only 283. Landsman approached the Haifa nurses with clear orders

> ...To make all possible efforts that not one baby reaching the age of two will abandon the center, but will immediately transfer to the Children-in-Passage Department. The success of operations in Jerusalem shows us that such action is possible if only there is devotion and interest on the part of the nurses.[409]

When children reached the age of four, it was customary to celebrate this landmark at a well-attended event — in the presence of parents, neighbors, public figures and members of the Hadassah Medical Federation. Landsman proposed the idea that the end of the four-year period during which children were under the supervision of the station for nursing babies and the Children-in-Passage Department be hallmarked by the Hadassah Medical Federation and cited in a festive gathering in which health certificates would be presented.

The first celebration of this kind was held in Jerusalem in April 1932 at Health Center A in the Old City; the format was subsequently adopted by all other Health Centers in the country the following year. Children were dressed in white, and each received a "health insignia" shaped like a Star of David emblazoned with the words "I'm Healthy." The Health Center was decorated for the occasion — an event that was honored by the presence of Henrietta Szold, who, according to one description, "gazed at the lovely tots continually, her eyes emanating light and much love through the hall."[410]

The official ceremony followed a set pattern. From eyewitness accounts of the content, one can savor the flavor of such celebrations. In one case, the nurse opened festivities, greeting the audience by declaring:

> *We have gathered together to celebrate a special festival — the festival of our children's maturation from nursing infants to toddlers...From here henceforth, our children have crossed the threshold into childhood, and this day is an important moment for both child and mother.*[411]

The nurse's greetings were followed by words of thanks from one of the mothers for the staff's dedicated care for their children. One such mother praised the staff, testifying:

> *Five times I gave birth in the Hadassah Hospital. The nurses helped me deliver for free or for a small sum. All five of my children received milk and clothing. The Almighty will bless you [the nurses] with long days and reward you for all your kindness and charitable deeds that you have done.*[412]

The nurses then summed up the four-year association with the Center, speaking of the importance of care that children had received at the Health Center, the significance of attending kindergarten, and the value of health and health education. The children received toothbrushes and Shemen™ toothpaste, and were granted health diplomas signed by the physician that hailed the mothers "for raising a healthy and handsome generation."[413]

One of the guests then numbered the attributes of the nurses' dedicated work. As was customary and in keeping with the tempo of the times in general, in one such case the delegate, a neighborhood elder, defined the nurses' role in historic — almost heroic — terms, categorized the staff at the Beit Yaakov Health Center as "...merciful nurses who partake in the rebirth of the [Jewish] People. Who care with love for the infants, in order to raise up a healthy and refreshing generation that will be the glory to its People and country."[414]

Festivities closed with a group photograph of nurses, mothers and children.

Work Principles

From the outset of its work in Eretz Israel, Hadassah set forth fundamental principles for its health education work and strictly followed them — without compromise. Kupat Holim and the Hebrew Women's Federation, who agreed to collaborate with Hadassah, were required to accept the work methods and principles set forth by Hadassah without question. Hadassah's activities were based on the following six principles:

Services in Health Centers provided gratis, open to all — regardless of religious or ethnic affiliation.

This "watchword" was reflected in the declaration of one of the nurses; Zelda Goldman, at a meeting of nurses in Haifa, stated emphatically: "It's an iron-clad rule with us: To receive anyone who turns to the Center, without distinction of class, ethnic group or race."[415]

Material assistance (milk, diapers and clothing) was provided only for needy mothers who came regularly to receive guidance and advice. As Hadassah's head nurse Bertha Landsman put it:

> *Our clinics are open to all expectant women and children, who wish to profit from education and guidance that our institutions can provide and we do not make any distinction between rich and poor. The Hadassah Medical Federation does not demand payment for its educational work.*[416]

Dr. Gruenfelder expressed similar sentiments:

> *Supervision is not influenced, neither by differences of social status of the Yishuv, nor by differences of education, nor by the cultural level of the parents. Supervision is a general question for the country that should not be viewed from a political or an economic viewpoint.*[417]

Work designed to educate the family regarding a healthy life and to instill a healthy lifestyle.

This approach was reflected in the protocols from a nurses' meeting in Haifa where it was stated clearly: "Public work in all places is conducted according to set principles whose basis is education of women and of the family as a whole."[418]

Uniform methods for care of infants at all Health Centers throughout the country.

Uniform methods were implemented for feeding (both nursing and with milk substitutes), clothing and diapering infants. Kupat Holim doctors collaborating with the Health Centers were required to work according to directives set by Hadassah medical staff.

Conduct of house visits as a core activity in overall programming.

Enhancing a uniform approach to care in the home among mothers throughout the country by public nurses was described as "a cornerstone of [Hadassah] work."[419] House visits were part and parcel of the environmental work of the Health Centers — an integral part of preventive medicine that allowed the staff to instill uniform methods throughout the country.

Health work encompassing the entire family.

Hadassah's work encompassed care of expectant mothers, new mothers after delivery, care of infants and care of "children-in-passage," kindergartners and schoolchildren. The entire family as a whole constituted a unit in itself, under the supervision of the nurse, who assessed the material, social and health status of the family through house visits.

Health work focused on the healthy child.

Health Centers did not engage in curative medicine — they did not receive sick children or distribute medications. As Landsman phrased it: "The password of our Health Centers is care of the healthy child."[420]

Indicative of this approach is a comment by Dr. Baruch Ostrovsky, a pediatrician who noted in his memoirs: "I maintained the hallowed principle not to provide [medical] treatment in *Tipat Chalav*."[421]

Indeed, in time, mothers came to understand that the purpose of the examination by a Health Center physician was not curative, but for advice and guidance only as to the general status and nutrition of their babies.

Difficulties in Application of Hadassah Principles

Health services on behalf of mothers and babies were one of the most outstanding branches of Hadassah's constructive work in Eretz Israel. The emphasis and centrality assigned to this work emanated from recognition of the fact that care for the health of mother and child was the foundation for a healthy population, and the basis for all medical work designed to enhance society. In application of its health education plans, Hadassah aspired to guide mothers in the raising of their children and to teach them healthy habits in order to both improve health and quality of life. Thus, there was much frustration in Hadassah circles when the staff found themselves confronted from the beginning with unexpected difficulties and numerous stumbling blocks on the path to realizing their plans.

Hadassah endeavors encountered six major obstacles in the implementation of their plans to enhance health and the quality of life in Eretz Israel.

1. Low attendance rates by mothers at Health Centers.

These customs were described in a report by Rachel Pesach, a nurse in the Tiberias Health Center whose account reflects the general milieu and folkways prevailing among mothers at the offset of services in Tiberias:

> *Rumors about the antics of the nurses spread by hearsay. "She" says to open the window. "She" says to remove the layer of dirt from the head — a shell thought by the masses to nurture the brain — particularly among Sephardic [Jewish] and Muslim ethnic groups. "She" bathed a two-week-old male child. And (what was illogical to these mothers), "she" says that it is necessary to nurse the child [only] every three hours. To accustom [the] mother to weigh the child was not easy. Belief in the evil eye worked against us and they have an explicit saying: "God does not bless it."*[422]

2. Difficulty accustoming mothers to the concept that the Health Centers were designed for healthy children only.

Mothers who brought their sick children to receive medical treatment were turned away, under the claim that the Health Center was designed for healthy babies. At the same time, mothers assumed that if their child was well, there was no reason to bring it to the center. To overcome this difficulty, the nurses promised mothers who came weekly for advice and guidance that they would receive all their child's basic needs gratis — diapers, sheets, clothing, bathing equipment and care.

3. Instilling the necessity of adopting an orderly feeding schedule.

The mothers refused to change their habits of nursing their infants every time they cried — day and night. The nurses taught them that feedings must be carried out every three hours by the clock, but the mothers continued to feed their children every time they cried, despite nurses' claims that this was detrimental to the child. Hedva Hilfer, a nurse at the Petach Tikva Health Center, wrote with marked frustration of this phenomenon: "[Mothers] relate to their children like a perpetual mobile that was always working — but only mouth-stomach, that always needs to eat, whenever the mother puts food in front of it."[423]

4. Difficulty in uprooting habits that were not suitable for the climate of Eretz Israel.

The nurses instructed mothers to dress their children in keeping with the seasons, fighting overdressing in winter and summer. Rachel Pesach wrote Henrietta Szold from Tiberias, a region on the Sea of Galilee afflicted by terribly hot summers:

> *How much we must, for instance, fight against excessive covering and wrapping, particularly in the summer. And these people [the religious **haredi**] have customs and habits from cold western countries so different from the Eretz Israel climate, that here in the summer these habits are the source of actual tragedies, particularly among tots. The excessive heat [has] results that are sometimes quite serious.*[424]

5. Lack of trust in the nurses.

The chief nurses in Hadassah-run Health Centers were in their mid-twenties, single and thus had not given birth themselves. Mothers refused to accept their instructions and in many cases listened only to the advice of the doctor. With time, the nurses succeeded in gaining their confidence that they — the nurses — could enhance the health of their children.

6. Lack of trust and cooperation among religious mothers.

Nurses complained that religious mothers were interested only in material assistance of milk and clothing, but were not interested in education or information that the nurses strove to pass on. Many families of Ashkenazi (i.e., European) origin living in poverty in residences supported by brethren from abroad — in the Old City in Jerusalem and adjacent neighborhoods such as Mea Shearim — did not bother to take their infants to the Health Center. Children-in-passage were not brought to the center because their mothers "pitied the time that would be wasted in lieu of Torah studies."[425] Expectant women also did not register with the center. Rachel Pesach, a nurse at one of the Jerusalem centers, wrote to Landsman to complain, clearly frustrated: "The Jewish *haredi* community is the most resistant...in accepting our influence in regard to amending and improving progressive hygiene rules for care of infants and children."[426]

She strove to influence them, but to no avail. The women adamantly refused to be swayed. Rachel Pesach and Leah Kleinmann claimed that the ultra-orthodox neighborhoods were heavily populated by families of Middle Eastern origin — from Iraq and Bukhara — whom, she commented, "came from the East, which is much more distanced from the influence of culture,"[427] while there was a lot more progress among those of European origin. In order to bridge the gap, the nurses conducted house visits among pregnant women, designed to convince them of the importance of consultation and medical supervision during pregnancy, but the women continued to refuse to comply.

Two primary reasons for their stubborn opposition were given. The first was a lack of faith in the advice offered, based on the claim that for generations they had raised and educated their children without an "infant nursing station" — reinforced by claims that "this is not a matter for deeply religious women."[428] The second was fear of the evil eye, which they believed could be aroused by the very act of weighing their babies.

Consequently, the nurses took a wise step to bring the ultra-orthodox women into their sphere of influence. They asked Dr. Yasski to mobilize the support of two leading and influential rabbinical authorities in Jerusalem religious circles — Rabbi Sonnenfeld and Rabbi Kook. They suggested that Dr. Yasski describe the important work being conducted by the Health Centers and the desire to help reduce infant mortality and enhance the health of women and new mothers, stressing that the sole goal was to educate toward physical health and teach fundamentals of preventive medicine. The two nurses suggested that the two rabbis be invited to visit the Health Centers to observe firsthand the work being done and the benefits gained by mother and child.

Dr. Yasski did write the two rabbis telling them of the special efforts being made by the Hadassah Medical Federation to establish a series of stations for infants and pregnant women throughout the country "in order to prevent illness."[429] In his endeavors to mobilize their support, Dr. Yasski chose his words accordingly, writing:

> ...There is nothing in this work detrimental to the Jewish faith, however much to our sorrow, we have encountered great difficulties in these endeavors, particularly among our **haredi** brethren. We understand that Your Honor understands and appreciates the value of this important work, particularly on behalf of our People who are weak and frail from two thousand years of adversity, and will willingly respond to our requests, and influence your community as much as you can, to help us in our war against disease.[430]

Dr. Yasski requested that the two rabbis explain at the synagogues "the value of preventing illness before it appears and the special importance of our institutions that are designed for this purpose."[431] Following the advice of the nurses, he invited them to visit the Health Centers, declaring: "...We are certain that you will be convinced just how much benefit is entailed in our work on behalf of our People today and in future generations."[432]

Despite examination of ongoing correspondence, no reference was found indicating that the rabbis indeed visited a Health Center, or even answered Dr. Yasski's letter; however, over the year's difficulties faced by the Health Centers in attracting members of the *haredi* community were mitigated. In the end, the religious population began to accept Hadassah's work, and the nurses eventually won high esteem among this community as well.

The difficulties that Hadassah encountered in its desire to introduce its educational-health program within the *haredi* community were reflected simply in the words of praise of one of the mothers, described in the report as "an Ashkenazi women of deep religious belief, the wife of a rabbi" who spoke in Yiddish at the ceremony for "children-in-passage" on behalf of the mothers at the Beit Yaakov Health Center:

I must admit in front of all the mothers and the nurses, that when I visited with my eldest son at the Center, I did not follow the instructions given to me by the nurses, and I had a lot of troubles. Now, Blessed be the Holy Name, my children are healthy and I am happy, because I have started doing everything as ordered and according to the advice of the nurses, and I am advising all mothers to visit the station.[433]

Thus, Hadassah encountered significant difficulties and strong opposition in carrying out its health-education program geared to provide progressive welfare services for "populations at risk." The organization's objectives, principles and methods were not readily accepted by the Yishuv in Eretz Israel, nor taken for granted as a natural and welcome progression. Acceptance by both European and Eastern communities could ultimately be gained only through unlimited perseverance, patience and persistence that eventually bore fruit.

From an historic viewpoint, the success of Hadassah's program constituted a genuine revolution in mother and child welfare in Eretz Israel during the Mandate period.

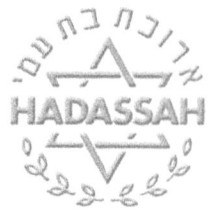

Chapter V

The Hadassah-Guggenheimer
Playgrounds Program

On the first day of September in 1925, the Old City of Jerusalem witnessed the opening of the first playground in Eretz Israel. This event was the first step in what was to become part of a general educational program for the establishment of playgrounds for the children of Eretz Israel, funded by Bertha Guggenheimer of Lynchburg, Virginia, and operated by the Hadassah American Zionist Women's Organization.

Soon after the foundation of the first playgrounds, training programs for counselors to operate them were developed and a national program for promoting the proper utilization of free time for children and youth took shape.

This chapter will discuss the establishment of the first three playgrounds in Eretz Israel during the British Mandate period. These playgrounds were founded on social and educational principles, and were among the first institutes of informal education in the country.[434] It was from these playgrounds that clubs, afternoon centers for schoolchildren, summer camps, and, finally, community centers developed.

What function did these playgrounds serve, and what were the forces that initiated them? This chapter focuses on the educational work carried out in the Guggenheimer-Hadassah playgrounds, examines their underlying principles, explains their unique significance in Eretz Israel during the British Mandate period, analyzes what part they played in the development of informal education in Eretz Israel and reveals the role Hadassah played in its formation.

Historical Background

Both the Balfour Declaration[435] and the conquest of Palestine by the British in late 1917 had significant political and economic repercussions on the status of the Yishuv. New players with new ideas entered the arena, established positions, undertook new initiatives and activities; these all affected the Jews in Eretz Israel.[436] It was during this time that Hadassah came to the aid of the Yishuv, leaving its mark on the development of educational and health services in Eretz Israel.

World War I left the Yishuv in Eretz Israel in a state of severe shortages and poor health. Of a population of 85,000 before the war, only 50,000 remained after expulsion, disease, epidemics, and death by starvation.[437] Those worse off by far were the children, primarily those who had survived the war years in the major cities. Constant hunger had damaged their health and development. According to Zalman Greenberg, the typhus epidemic of 1916–1917 among the Jewish population of Jerusalem had struck hardest at adults, leaving many orphans behind.[438]

In 1918, a delegation of the World Zionist Organization (WZO), headed by Dr. Chaim Weizmann, obtained permission from the British government to come to the country. The delegation was shocked by conditions in the Yishuv, and decided to organize emergency aid in order to rehabilitate and reorganize its institutions. A significant part of the task of rehabilitation was given to the American Zionist Organization. The responsibility for this rehabilitation was then transferred to Hadassah, which was already involved in philanthropic efforts in Eretz Israel.

Hadassah had been founded in 1912, with the aim of improving education, health, hygiene, and sanitation in Eretz Israel. Philanthropy and Zionism were the two main tenets of the organization, and, as David Ben-Gurion once said, "it is hard to tell whether they are more philanthropic or more Zionist."[439] From 1918 through 1921, Hadassah was active mainly in organizing aid for the Yishuv in Eretz Israel through the auspices of the WZO, and in establishing welfare services.[440] Health services were provided primarily by the American Zionist Medical Unit (the Unit),[441] which acted under the aegis of Hadassah, but which was actually a separate entity. In 1921, the Unit, which had originally been a temporary organization, became the autonomous Hadassah Medical Organization, which would from then on function on a permanent basis in Eretz Israel.

The main focus of Hadassah activity was the Jewish population of Jerusalem, which had suffered more during the war than any other Jewish population center in Eretz Israel, primarily because of poor living conditions, severe overcrowding, and greater financial dependence on economic aid from Diaspora Jewish communities. This financial aid had ceased with the outbreak of World War I, which led to a crisis situation for the residents of the city.

Out of 45,000 Jewish residents of Jerusalem on the eve of the war, only 26,000 remained, and the number of orphaned children was particularly high. Many of these children wandered the streets of the city, with nowhere to go and no one, not even an educational-institutional framework, to care for them. In a few instances, they even "died in the street," as noted by Eliezer Hoffein[442] in one of his reports on the state of Jewish orphans in Jerusalem. According to Hoffein, in 1918 there were nearly 3,000 children in Jerusalem who had no father to support them.[443] Rehabilitating the city's residents, particularly the children, was the top priority for the Unit and Hadassah.

In the summer of 1925, philanthropist Bertha Guggenheimer visited Jerusalem with her niece, Irma Lindheim, who would later become president of Hadassah (1926–1928). From Lynchburg, Virginia, Bertha Guggenheimer (1847–1927) took special interest in and supported a number of organizations, among them the Red Cross and the National Playground and Recreation Association of America; she was a member of the latter. Her interest in the recreation movement began in 1912, in the wake of a congress on recreation held in the city of her birth, Richmond, Virginia. One year later, she established the Playground and Recreation Association of her hometown of Lynchburg, and served as its president until it became one of the departments of the Lynchburg municipality. She established the city's first playground, called the "Guggenheimer-Milliken Playground," after her daughter Celeste Milliken. As she was a pioneer in championing playgrounds in Lynchburg, she was known as "the mother of playgrounds."[444]

Both Guggenheimer and her niece were stunned by the circumstances of the children of Jerusalem, particularly those who lived in the Old City. Children and teenagers wandering through the streets, throwing stones, playing cards, sitting idly in Arab cafes, or searching through garbage heaps were a common sight in the Old City. Guggenheimer realized immediately that if children and youths were to be prevented from wandering around aimlessly after school hours, there was an urgent need for playgrounds staffed, supervised and directed by counselors or teachers and health workers. The execution of this plan was handed over to Hadassah.

The Evolution of the Playground

The playgrounds, whose fundamental premise was to offer free play and various sports and social activities, were erected in the crowded neighborhoods settled by the poor in industrial cities during the nineteenth century. Their aim was to occupy children and teenagers during their leisure time and to teach them to plan their free time effectively and enjoyably. Thus, they shaped each child's behavioral patterns in a way essential for improving quality of life.

The pioneer of the modern playground was Robert Owen. A British industrialist and humanitarian, Owen founded near his factory a playground for children aged three and over. He called the institution an "infant school," and in it provided informal education for children, with an emphasis on health and athletic activity. Later, additional institutions would be established throughout England and France, based on the same format.[445] By the turn of the century, playgrounds were very common across England, and their main purpose was to "get the children off the streets." Playgrounds were erected in every neighborhood, and equipped with swings and climbing frames; they also offered activities such as carpentry and other crafts. Extensive educational-social activity was also held there, under the guidance of counselors.

In the United States, the first playgrounds for children and teenagers were established at the end of the nineteenth century by Joseph Lee, who saw them as a means of both preventing delinquency and educating youth.[446] The phenomenon of children idly loitering or playing in the busy streets — and causing more than a few traffic accidents — provided additional impetus for creating a safe place to play. As the playground culture became well established in the United States, the Playground Association of America was founded in 1906; it was the first organization of its kind in the world.

Playgrounds in Eretz Israel

The first move in establishing playgrounds in Eretz Israel was that of Guggenheimer during her visit to Eretz Israel in the summer of 1925. With the help of the Local Board, Guggenheimer found a lot at the edge of the Jewish Quarter in the Old City of Jerusalem and equipped it with playground apparatus like that found in the United States. Thus, on September 1, 1925, the Sha'ar Zion Playground, the first ever in Eretz Israel, opened to the public, under the direction of Lillian Kornfeld. In the years that followed, additional playgrounds were established in Jerusalem, and these were directed by Rachel Schwartz,[447] who would eventually be appointed superintendent of the playground project. These playgrounds were operated by a staff of counselors that Schwartz had trained.[448]

The playground was a kind of neighborhood club, a place where children and teenagers could spend their leisure hours, all year long, in recreational, play, movement, and creative activities. The implementation of educational principles inculcated diverse patterns of activity in the children, helped consolidate groups of children of similar ages through play, and helped encourage neighborhood and community organization.[449]

The playground included an expansive space with enough room for games involving movement, a play area with apparatus and sports equipment, and a clubhouse building where educational-cultural activities were held. An extensive recreational program was also offered, which included drama, carpentry, games, singing, sculpting, and instruction in playing musical instruments, drawing, and crafts.

The playground activity was organized and executed according to an educational program, planned in advance by the playground director and the counselors. They were assisted by the Advisory Board, headed by Moshe Shvabe.[450] The goals of the playgrounds established by Shvabe included: Instructing the child in the proper use of free time, and training him for the leisure culture; organizing teenagers who had not joined one of the youth movements; preventing loitering, neglect, and delinquency among school dropouts; and preparing young people for life in the working society of the Yishuv in Eretz Israel.

The initial aim of the playgrounds in the Old City of Jerusalem was to keep children away from the harmful influence of the street, to give them a respite from their difficult living conditions, and to bring them into a warm, sympathetic, educationally and culturally healthy environment. Two years after its establishment, the playground was moved to a larger lot next to Zion Gate.[451] This move was also funded by Guggenheimer, but she never got a chance to see the new playground. In her will, she set up a special fund for the erection and maintenance of playgrounds.[452] The trustees[453] appointed Hadassah as executor; the organization took upon itself all responsibility for the enterprise, which from then on was called the Guggenheimer-Hadassah Playgrounds.

Hadassah participation in the playground program was a natural act. From its early years, Hadassah championed the message calling for "establishing a new generation, healthy in body and mind" in Eretz Israel and focused its activity mainly on improving the health and welfare of the young generation, recognizing that addressing the health needs of the child was the foundation for a healthy society. Thus, Hadassah planned and implemented a comprehensive public health program for Jewish children in Eretz Israel in the realm of preventive medicine. The program included the establishment of Mother & Child Health Centers, known as *Tipat Chalav,* setting in place school-based health and hygiene services, organizing a "cafeteria fund" to provide school lunch programs, and building playgrounds for children and youth for extracurricular activities. The slogan "to bring up a new generation, health in body and mind" was not just the objective of the Zionist Movement — it was also one of the deepest aspirations of pioneers in education in Eretz Israel. They saw their role as educators of the new generation growing up in Mandate Palestine, and viewed their work not only in terms of Hebrew-national education and inculcation of the Hebrew language as the mother tongue of native sons and daughters; they also considered it their duty to maintain their students' good health. This ranged from care for students' well being and inculcating proper health and hygienic habits, to information about contagious diseases (malaria, trachoma, ringworm), understanding disease factors and preventive measures students should take. All this was carried out based on a deep concern for the health of the child as the foundations for creating a strong and healthy new generation.

Already in the founding convention of the Teachers' Federation in Eretz Israel held in 1903, it was decided that parallel to regular subjects — Bible, science, nature, social studies, current events, etc. — the curriculum would include hygiene, gymnastics, music and art, "as is customary in all the progressive schools of enlightened peoples." The objective of gymnastics was to promote "physical fitness and steadfastness of purpose (*koach ratzon*)" — objectives that reflected broader aspects of Jewish national awakening that encouraged concern for one's body as an important element in the Zionist national revival and deepening one's ties to Eretz Israel. A central motif was that physical revival goes hand-in-hand with national revival — forging a "New Jew" who would lead a national Zionist revolution in Jewish life. The model of the New Jew was the antithesis of perceptions of the Diaspora Jew. Such New Jews would be proud, confident and endowed with physical and spiritual stamina.[454]

The Educational Work Program of Eretz Israel's Playgrounds

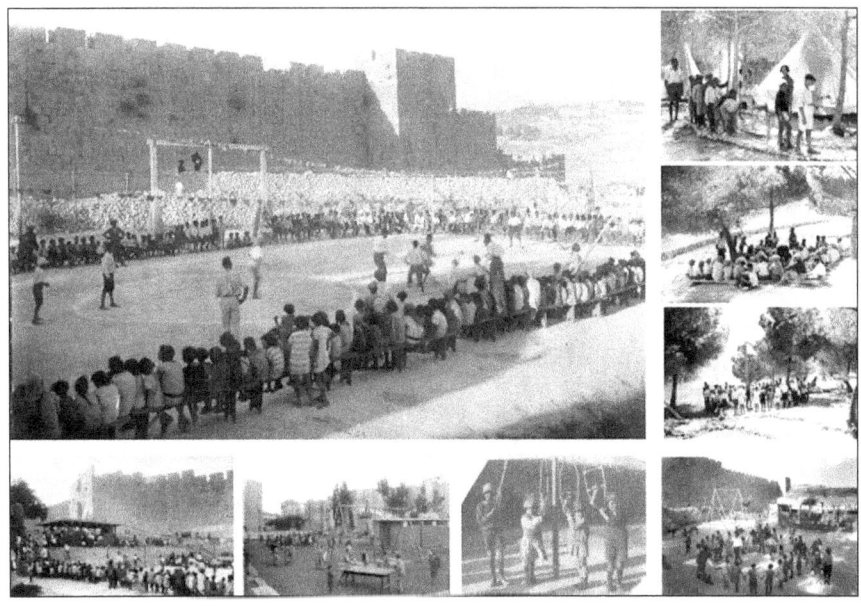

The Hadassah-Guggenheimer Playgrounds in Jerusalem 1920s-1940s (Courtesy of Rothschild-Hadassah Archives, Jerusalem).

The goal of the playgrounds was to add content and interest to the leisure time of the child, and to educate him to utilize this time as effectively and enjoyably as possible. The playgrounds were erected near the neighborhood schools, or even inside them. This proximity to the schools was mutually advantageous; the playgrounds benefited from economic savings and the use of classrooms, bathrooms, and the schoolyard during after-school hours. The schools, on the other hand, permitted their pupils to use the playground equipment —

i.e., swings, ladders, and, after their installation, showers — during school hours.

In February 1929, another playground was opened in the *Kol Israel Haverim* (Alliance) School, in the Machane Yehuda neighborhood of Jerusalem's New City.[455] The counselors who were sent to staff the new playground encouraged the local children to come and join in the activities; they invited the older girls to help decorate it and get ready for the opening celebration. Word spread like wildfire, and on the very first day it opened, hundreds of children "hungry for play" showed up.

The playground's opening became possible only after negotiations between Dr. Ephraim Bluestone,[456] director of Hadassah, and Yitzhak Bassan, the principal of the *Kol Israel Haverim* (Alliance) School. In a letter sent on July 17, 1928, Dr. Bluestone explained the intentions of the Playground Department of the Hadassah Medical Organization to expand its works and to establish more playgrounds in Jerusalem, in addition to the one next to Zion Gate in the Old City:

> *It has been proposed that the present program of work in the playgrounds be expanded, in order to include various educational activities, particularly instruction in personal hygiene. The Jerusalem Playground Committee has scouted out a number of locations and, thanks to the generosity of C. B., has examined the option of putting the yard of the school under his direction to such a purpose. It has been concluded that this is the most suitable location, for the following reasons: a) the lot is located next to a well-maintained school, with a competent administration; b) the lot is large enough for the purpose to which it will be put; c) the lot is near crowded neighborhoods populated by poor Jews. After serious consideration of all possibilities available to us, the said committee has decided to enter into negotiation with C.B. with the aim of establishing a playground in the yard of his school. It is understood that this arrangement will not require any additional expense on your part. The pupils of your school will be able to use the part of the lot that you put at our disposal during school hours. ...We hereby are sending a copy of this letter to Mrs.*

Schwartz, Playground Superintendent, who will approach C.B. in order to clarify any remaining details with him.[457]

The *Kol Israel Haverim* School benefited from the experience that had been gained with its two predecessors, and it was a resounding triumph. In the words of playground counselor Rachel HaMeirit-Gorodisky, it became an "empire."[458] In the wake of its success, additional playgrounds based on the same format were established throughout Eretz Israel: in Tel Aviv, Rechovot, Gedera, Ekron, Nes Ziona, Rishon LeZion, Tiberias, and even the newly settled villages and farms.[459]

The playground at the *Kol Israel Haverim* School in Jerusalem, which the children called *Kikar HaNoar* (Youth Square), attracted many children from the Machane Yehuda neighborhood, which was located at the center of a poor Jewish area in the New City of Jerusalem. The playground included a large inner courtyard, where American-style playground equipment was installed, and a large hall. In the hall, different social and cultural activities were held; there were "corners" for drawing, crafts, carpentry, music, drama, sports, camping, nature, dance, and basket weaving. The activities were open to all the children, and each child was free to choose what he wanted to do. In the outdoor play area, various movement and social games were offered.

Special activities were also available, such as excursions and camping trips and other special projects. Some of these projects were erecting a meteorology station, putting together a museum from the children's collections, keeping small animals and maintaining a garden, and organizing book fairs for National Book Week. As Rachel Schwartz put it, "...in order to satisfy all types of children of all ages, a broad and diverse program was required. We must diversify the program to such an extent that every child will be able to find what he wants to do, as well as show him new sources of satisfaction to which he has not yet been exposed."[460]

Some 300–400 children aged three to sixteen participated in the activity offered by the playgrounds — an average of 200 every day.

The girls and boys were divided into groups, and each group had its own counselor. The playground counselors were young teachers specializing in youth education. The staff was reinforced by teacher trainees from the Mizrachi Teachers' Seminar for Girls, who were encouraged to participate by their school director.

The Children's Council worked alongside the counselors. Children's Council members were elected by the children, and met on a weekly basis. Its main function was to solve immediate problems of order, discipline, and supervision, and to take part in preparing and executing activity programs. The idea of establishing the Children's Council was put forward by Schwartz; according to her, "in order for the children to manage things, they must be involved in formulating its values."[461]

The scouting movement also assisted with the activity in the playground, and its help was gratefully accepted by both the staff and the children. Every day two Scout leaders came to help the staff with the implementation of the pedagogic program. Despite their youth, the Scouts carried out their commitments with a large measure of success, earning the admiration of the smaller children in particular, who did not hide their dream of being Scout leaders when they grew up.

The playground opened at three o'clock in the afternoon and its activities continued until six. At first, the children engaged as they wished in individual activity in the different activity "corners." Afterwards, a general activity was held for all the children. The minutes of one meeting show proposals for appropriate concluding activities to end each day: Sunday, a story and play; Monday, a film; Tuesday, collective play; Wednesday, a concert; Thursday, a general discussion; and for the Sabbath, a ceremony.[462]

After the younger children were sent home, with the catchphrase *"pea'al ve'sameach"* ("play and be happy"), activities for the older children began. These included talks, discussions on current events, and social games, and continued until seven in the evening. According to Malka and Yosef Koriel, who as children came regularly to the Machane Yehuda Playground, special attention was devoted to the older children; they helped the counselors carry out the pedagogic program, and also formed the nucleus of the group of future counselors.

At the initiation of Baruch Ben-Ishai, head counselor, special activities were organized for the older group and their unique areas of interest. Ben-Ishai understood the needs of the older children, and invited youth leaders from the Scouts and the *Machanot Olim* (Immigrants' Camps) and *HaNoar Ha'Oved* (Working Youth) youth movements to talk with them about their activities, in order to help them make decisions about their future. Some of the older children trained to be playground counselors, and others joined the *Haganah* (Defense) organization. It was in just this way that Malka Koriel began working as a counselor for groups of young people in the Makor Baruch neighborhood — where the activities of the Machane Yehuda Playground had been transferred — and continued to do so until she became pregnant. Koriel and her husband Yosef had met at the playground, and were even married there. Their wedding was held in a shed at the Makor Baruch Playground, surrounded by children, counselors, and a delegation of Hadassah women.[463]

> *An Annual Review of the Guggenheimer-Hadassah Playgrounds informed that over the course of a year (January 1933 to January 1934) five Guggenheimer playgrounds were opened in Palestine: two in Jerusalem (at Har Zion and Machane Yehuda), one in Tel Aviv, one in Haifa, and one in Safed. "The number of children visiting these five playgrounds on an average day is 607. ...*[464]

In 1939, the first and the only playground of its kind in the Kibbutz Movement was established at Kibbutz Mishmar Ha'Emek. The Mishmar Ha'Emek Playground was identical to the playgrounds established in the cities and operated according to the principle stated by Bertha Guggenheimer: that the playground should be open to children and teenagers of all ethnic groups and nationalities, regardless of religion, race, or gender. This project was initiated by Irma Lindheim, Guggenheimer's niece, who received support from the Guggenheimer Fund. Arrangements were made for regular visits by Arab children from the surrounding area. When the members of Hadassah came to visit Lindheim at Mishmar Ha'Emek, they saw Guggenheim's vision in action: Children of all ages played happily together, without regard to religion, race, or nationality. The playground was opened daily to the use of the kibbutz children, but the Arab children from the neighborhood could visit it only on certain days and during certain hours. Its activity, as in the other mixed Arab–Jewish playgrounds, was based mainly on physical activity of all kinds.

Principles of the Playgrounds in Eretz Israel

Equality for All

The primary directive underlying the operation of the playgrounds was that they be open to children and teenagers of all ethnic groups and nationalities, regardless of religion, race, or gender. The first playground, established in a mixed Arab–Jewish neighborhood in the Old City of Jerusalem, was an innovation, because it was the first educational framework of its type established in Eretz Israel with the aim of providing educational–social activity for children regardless of race, religion, or nationality, as dictated both by Guggenheimer in her will, and by Hadassah ideology.

Admirable as it was, this principle generated many unexpected difficulties. The playgrounds were erected in a mixed environment, whose population included both Arabs and Jews of all kinds: Sephardic and Ashkenazi, secular and religious. Kornfeld related that

> Most of the children were of Sephardic extraction, and these were the first to come in large numbers to the playground. The Arab children were in the minority, and therefore they were afraid of the Jewish children. It was a source of great satisfaction for me to see Jewish and Arab children playing happily together.[465]

Be that as it may, the playground activity also increased the friction between Jews and Arabs, and between secular and religious Jews.

Jewish–Arab Relations

The first playground, Har Zion (from here on referred to as Har Zion A), which was established in 1925, hosted many Jewish children. The Arab children, who were in the minority, were afraid of them, and hesitant to play with them. The second playground, Har Zion B, which opened in 1927, was located in a poor Arab area, and Armenian and Arab children made up some 60% of all the children who came to play there.[466]

Therefore, special educational efforts were demanded on the part of the counselors to overcome the language difficulties and differences in mentality.

Organized group social games and schoolyard games occupied a central place in programming of outdoors activities due to their educational value and their ability to contribute to improving relationships between children from different ethnic backgrounds. Due to different mentalities and linguistic barriers, the instructors abstained from conducting activities based on reading or dramatizing stories or discussions of current events. Through shared games Christian, Muslim and Jewish children learned the importance of cooperating in social life and interacting on a social level beyond the limitations of language.

Additionally, the playground served as a bridge between the rich Arab children and the children of the poor Arabs, who were compelled by circumstances to play together and participate in the collective playground.

In Schwartz's words, "...it was good to see Jewish, Muslim, and Christian children playing together, in friendship, in the very same place where these same children used to throw stones at each other."[467] Schwartz related that in such unique circumstances, it was difficult to speak only Hebrew: "I had to plan [the work program] so that no Arab child would be forced to learn Hebrew, and so that every child would feel comfortable — the program had to suit all, not only the athletic, but also the handicapped, regardless of religion or nationality."[468] Often, the situation became absurd; Schwartz described an instance in which she addressed an Arab boy with "*Kef hallak?"* (Arabic for "How are you?") only to have him reply, *"Baruch Hashem"* (Hebrew for "Fine, thank G-d").

At the second convention of the counselors of the Guggenheimer-Hadassah Playgrounds in Eretz Israel, held at the Machane Yehuda Playground, December 30 through 31, 1932, Counselor Miriam Allouf told of her difficulties in working with Arabs, who constituted a significant percentage of the children playing at the Har Zion B Playground. She suggested hiring an Arab counselor to work with the Arab children. This proposal, however, was deemed impractical, because of the difficulty involved in finding someone appropriate for the task. It was decided that the matter would be handled by a special committee that would discuss ways of working together with the Arab population.[469]

The minutes of the Advisory Board of the Guggenheimer-Hadassah Playgrounds showed that that the Har Zion B playground posed particular difficulties because of the way in which the work was done there, and the possibility of moving the Jewish children elsewhere and leaving the playground to the Arab children was discussed. Henrietta Szold, then director of the Department of Social Work of the National Council, objected to this solution, claiming that the playground was of great political value in creating understanding and tolerance between the two populations, "as Hadassah made its rule never to distinguish between Arab and Jew."[470] It should be noted that the Jewish–Arab issue was a permanent part of the Hadassah's creed, at the behest of the organization's founder, Szold, who since her emigration to Eretz Israel in 1920 had supported organizations advocating Jewish–Arab outreach, such as *Brith Shalom* (Peace Covenant).[471]

Being practical, Szold proposed placing the question before the Jewish Agency and the members of *Brith Shalom*, noting that if a decision was reached to establish separate playgrounds, conditions should be determined for the playground's transfer to Arab hands, and the National Council should be able to ensure that it was being used solely for the purpose for which it was established. However, Libbie Berkson, one of the members of the Advisory Board, claimed that she was certain that "Mrs. Guggenheimer would not have given any money to a non-integrated playground, and thus the playground must be open to both Jewish and Arab children. Therefore, the playground should be moved somewhere else with more Jewish children and fewer Arab children."[472] In the end, the Advisory Board supported maintaining a joint playground for Jews and Arabs, and decided that the present playground would be moved to a safer and more appropriate place in the Old City, with fewer Arabs, conveniently located for children of all religions.[473]

The "mixed" playground aroused the opposition of the neighborhood residents, both Jewish and Arab. Some even intervened in the social activity held in the playground, and made critical remarks to the staff. Schwartz, the playground director, occasionally heard Arab passers-by comment that the playground should be burned down; no less blatant criticism could also be heard from Jews. Schwartz went to the nurse of the neighborhood *Tipat Chalav* station, and asked her to tell the Jewish mothers to send their children to the playground. However, the nurse told her, "I can't do that! I myself [am] against it, and I wouldn't send my children there!"[474]

One of the playground's Arab neighbors, Arif Pasha, did much to help the playground staff in all issues connected to the children's "education"; however, he also intervened frequently in their quarrels, and to Schwartz's disapproval, he went so far as to punish them. She was forced to ask him "to limit his involvement." Schwartz did use Arif Pasha's educational advice on at least one memorable occasion. One Sabbath, when she was leaving the playground, she met an Arab boy named Saliman who told her that a gang of Jewish girls had closed in on him when he came to the playground, shouting that the Mufti should be slaughtered, and all Arabs killed. Schwartz felt as if she was to blame, but took the opportunity to repeat what Arif Pasha often said: "Time heals all." Arif Pasha said this whenever he encountered Arab and Jewish children shouting insults at each other.

In contrast with the adults, who accepted the playgrounds with suspicion, the children — who lived in poverty and shortage, without toys, and without appropriate places to play — needed little urging to come and play. A swing was enough to win them over. Indeed, after a few months of joint activity, harmony did flourish among the children.

The organized social games were a central part of the playground activity program, due to both their great educational value and their significant contribution to improving relations between the children from different ethnic groups. Christian, Muslim, and Jewish children learned the importance of cooperation in daily life in society, beyond language limitations, from their experience in the playgrounds. It may be said that this was the first attempt to foster successful social relations between Jews and Arabs under appropriate supervision, which in itself was truly innovative in Eretz Israel at that time

The problem of relations between Jews and Arabs occupies a special place in American Zionism. From the 1920s onward, various Zionist organizations demonstrated special sensitivity toward this problem, but particularly the largest American-Jewish Zionist organization — Hadassah. This topic was given special emphasis in Hadassah's platform. The moving force behind this approach was Szold, one of the founders of Hadassah, who inspired and championed its adoption. From the time of her own immigration to Eretz Israel in 1920, Szold showed particular affection for organizations that considered bringing Jews and Arabs closer together to be one of their prime objectives: *Brith Shalom* (Peace Covenant), *Kedma Mizracha* (Eastward), *HaLiga leHitkarvut Yehudit-Aravit* (the League for Jewish-Arab Rapprochement) and *Ichud* (Union). Under the influence of these organizations Szold supported the establishment of a bi-national state in Eretz Israel. Hadassah did not embrace this vision of Szold's emphatically or fully, but nevertheless, the organization was deeply involved in promoting Jewish and Arab fraternity.[475] Only slowly and gradually did the organization, in the latter part of 1942, come to recognize and support the establishment of a Jewish state in the Eretz Israel, although even after this point, Hadassah continued to belong to the "moderate" stream within American Zionism on this issue.

During the 1920s and 1930s, there was a group of very influential women among the Hadassah leadership who held key positions in the organizations and who supported the vision of a bi-national state. They proposed Jewish initiatives to develop ties of mutual understanding between the peoples in areas of mixed Jewish-Arab settlement in domains where Hadassah operated: health projects, infant houses and playgrounds.[476]

Irma Lindheim — Hadassah president, 1926–1928 — endeavored, in practice, to establish ties between Jewish and Arab children. She partook in the establishment of a playground in the Old City of Jerusalem that served both Jewish and Arab children, and in 1938 a similar project in Kibbutz Mishmar Ha'Emek in the Jezreel Valley was embarked on that included regular visits to the playground by children from surrounding Arab villages.

Establishment of "mixed playgrounds" generated apprehension, reservations and outright opposition among adults, Jewish and Arab parents alike. But the children integrated swiftly and well in educational activities. The playgrounds attracted public figures who came to observe the "miraculous coexistence" exhibited by the Jewish and Arab children, how the children played naturally with other children oblivious of the ethnic and religious differences that set them apart.[477] In normal times, the atmosphere on the Har Zion Playgrounds was good, but in "stormy times" sensitivities heightened, and occasionally it was necessary to close the playground for short periods until things subsided. Thus was the case during the 1929 Arab Riots, beginning on August 23[478] and lasting a week; in the wake of the riots, the playground was closed for two and a half months until things settled down.[479] When it was reopened the number of children who came the first day was small, primarily due to fear, hostility and hatred that had not dissipated. Yet, the first day passed tranquilly and the impression was that things were back on keel, but the next day playground instructors found graffiti on the gate saying "Down with the Balfour Declaration — Down with the Jews." Schwartz, who was responsible for the playgrounds, sent a report to the Guggenheimer Playground Committee in America, which was underwriting the program, in which she described the impact of the 1929 Arab Riots on playground operations. She cited that educational considerations were what led her to re-open the playground and not political considerations, and that the playground was the first among educational institutions in the Old

City that had returned to normal operation, despite fears that this would expose the children and the instructors to possible harm, citing that in her opinion it was important to demonstrate no signs of weakness to Arab neighbors.[480]

The presence of Jewish and Arab children on the playground continued to be small for a number of months due to parental objections. One of the Arabs sent an article to the newspapers in which he took to task one of his Arab neighbors who in the past had volunteered at the playground, charging that he had shown friendship toward the instructors, calling him with derision "a Zionist." There were cases of violence among the children themselves, as well. An Arab youth of 14, who had been removed from the playground for failure to follow the rules, assembled some 30 Arab youth and organized a demonstration across from the playground. The teens blocked the gate and did not permit the instructors to leave, while shouting, "Butcher the Jews!" The situation calmed down and quiet was restored only after the police intervened.

A year after the riots, the situation still had not improved. The atmosphere in the neighborhood was tense, some Jewish families left the Old City and the number of children visiting the playground remained low. The advisory council called a special meeting to discus the future of the Har Zion Playgrounds. Among those present were Szold and Dr. Chaim Yasski, the director of Hadassah Hospital. It was decided to close the playground despite arguments that it was important from a political standpoint to continue its operation. Other participants in the meeting argued that there was no justification for putting the safety of the children in jeopardy to advance the playground's educational goals.[481]

In keeping with Hadassah's ideological outlook and according to Guggenheimer's will, which donated money to create mixed playgrounds, the members of Hadassah felt that they should continue to nurture the concept of mixed playgrounds despite the many difficulties encountered in actually operating them and the opposition encountered among the adult population. Thus, a second mixed playground was established in 1936 in Tel Aviv, but it was also received with mixed feelings and did not gain the support of parents. The atmosphere at the playground was influenced by the political-security situation in Eretz Israel at the time —

the 1936–1939 Arab Revolt[482] that broke out soon after the playground was built. Activities on the playground were limited and even ceased for brief periods. Re-openings were accompanied, each time, by parental objections, protesting vigorously against opening the playground and claiming they didn't want their daughters "to mix with Arab children."[483] Following intervention by the Municipality, the playground was opened on an experimental footing, but this time only boys — Jewish and Arab — were permitted to enter. Difficulties continued to accompany this playground, and after a portion of the members of the Tel Aviv playground committee didn't support the mixed playground concept, it was decided to close the playground and Hadassah decided to establish another one in a mixed neighborhood in Jaffa — the main objective being not to abandon the vision of mixed playgrounds.[484]

Secular–Religious Relations

The problem of relations between secular and religious Jews greatly concerned the pedagogic staff of the two Har Zion playgrounds and the Machane Yehuda Playground. This issue was the root of the friction between the playgrounds and the local residents. Playground activity took place five days a week, Sunday through Thursday, and Sabbaths and holidays; in addition, on the Sabbath there were always joint activities for children and parents. Soccer and other games were organized, and 300–400 children and family members participated. This meant that the playgrounds became active neighborhood recreation centers.

Rachel HaMeirit-Gorodisky, a counselor at the Har Zion and Machane Yehuda playgrounds, related that the Sabbath activities were carefully planned so as not to desecrate the Sabbath: "It was wonderful for the children, because they were idle, they had nowhere to play at home, no yard, and no toys, and the playground occupied them and gave them something interesting to do during the afternoon hours, all week long and on the Sabbath as well."[485] Yitzhak Nesher, who directed the first playground in Rechovot, which was established in 1932, said that the Sabbaths were a resounding success; more than 150 children and their parents, from all over the area, came on that day, while during the week only 60 children on average showed up per day.[486]

The rabbis and the religious establishment objected strongly to the Sabbath activity, and the religious public sharply criticized it. Particularly interesting was the attitude of the children who attended *heder* (traditional Jewish elementary school) toward the idea of spending free time at the playground in general, and playing games in particular. They came regularly to the playground, only to stand outside the fence watching the children playing and spending time unproductively. Kornfeld told that one day two five-year-old *heder* children came to the Har Zion A Playground to watch the children at play with disdain. In response to her question as to why they did not join the children, the two laughed and said, "We're not like them." When she sought to find out what exactly they meant by this, they explained, "Those are children who play, but we are children who study."[487] However, very gradually, natural instinct overcame their superiority, and these two children joined in the games. Kornfeld watched them at play; they swung on swings for the first time in their lives, and were so terrified when their feet left the ground that she felt real compassion for them.

As mentioned, in early 1929 the playground in the Machane Yehuda neighborhood was opened. It immediately aroused hostility on the part of the local residents, both secular and religious. The playground was located next to the Etz Chaim Talmud Torah yeshiva, whose director objected to the activities held there; he claimed that according to Biblical law, it was a sin for girls and boys to play together. According to Schwartz, the director of the yeshiva was enraged because his pupils could not concentrate on the Talmud, and instead of keeping their eyes on their books stole furtive looks at the boys and girls at play.[488] He demanded that the playground be closed. However, Schwartz told him, "Our children have a natural instinct to play. How can a rabbi deny it?"[489] Because she declined to do as he asked, the yeshiva director prosecuted her, and she received an order from the Rabbinical Court to appear before it and explain why she would not close the playground. Sorrowfully, Schwartz turned to the Chief Ashkenazi Rabbi of the Yishuv in Eretz

Israel, Rabbi Abraham Yitzhak Kook[490] — the same rabbi Dr. Yasski turned to for help when faced with *haredi* opposition to hygienic and health advice. "Daughter," Rabbi Kook told her, "attend to your work, and all will be well."[491]

It was no accident that Schwartz went to Rabbi Kook for assistance. Since his first appointment, as the rabbi of the city of Jaffa, Rabbi Kook had criticized traditional *haredi* (ultra-Orthodox) education and supported the development of modern national religious education. He encouraged sports activities and spoke highly of instruction in exercise and art education. In his words, "we need a healthy body...we have neglected physical health and valor."[492] Rabbi Kook's withdrawal of the objection was in keeping with his outlook, particularly his position on health education, and was in line with his view that "new foundations must be built for the relationship between *haredim* [religious men] and free men, where the old will be renewed and the new will become sanctified."[493]

In addition, Rabbi Kook's support of the playground encouraged the playground's counselors to organize a summer playground for children from the *haredi* community. The minutes of the board meetings of the Guggenheimer-Hadassah Playgrounds show that this initiative was accepted by the *haredi* community, based on the principle that only ultra-orthodox children would attend it and the activity would be set according to their religious tradition. Ben-Ishai, who was appointed as the regional superintendent of playgrounds, said in a report on the summer playgrounds for the *haredi* children that

> *More than one hundred children participated and the activities were highly successful. This was the first time that we had managed to reach these sectors of the population, and it was a very valuable experience. Since some surplus remained in the Agudat Ysrael budget, and in the operating budget of the Guggenheimer Fund, it was decided to extend the summer playground for the **haredi** children, which had been so successful, for another week, in addition to the original two months.*[494]

The neutral position of the playground enterprises with regard to secular-religious relations was put to the test when children from families that had converted to Christianity under the influence of the Christian Mission wanted to join in the activities. The playground staff accepted those children, allowing them to participate in playground activities. Kornfeld noted in her reports that in one instance, a group of children helped a 15-year-old girl whose parents had converted, and encouraged her to continue to come to the playground. The Scouting Movement counselors who helped operate the playground accepted this girl as a member of one of their groups, and even managed to find her a job with a Jewish family.

Medical Supervision

Hadassah's medical and health education supervision was another principle underpinning the operation of the playgrounds. One of the first steps of Hadassah in Eretz Israel was to take responsibility for medical care in all the schools and kindergartens of the Board of Education, and to establish a Department of School Hygiene. This was the first of many preventive medicine enterprises, in accordance with Hadassah's major aim: raising a new generation, healthy in mind and body. Dr. Mordechai Berachiahu, head of the School Hygiene Department, said, "This is a difficult task in Eretz Israel, where customs, tradition, and way of life differ from one street to the next and from one neighborhood to the next."[495]

The playgrounds were also under the supervision of Dr. Berachiahu's Department. One problem, raised in a meeting of school doctors and nurses headed by Dr. Berachiahu, was that the children came to the playground at three in the afternoon, and due to the "physical play," became overtired. The teachers then complained that the children were fatigued the next day at school, which interfered with their studies.[496] It was decided to formulate a recommendation that the playgrounds be opened at four o'clock, that shelter from the sun would be provided, that space be set aside for rest, and that the children be supervised by someone "with an understanding of children's hygiene in general, and of exercise in particular."

The playgrounds were open to all children, but in order to participate in social activities the children had to undergo eye and skin examinations every three months. Children found to be infected with trachoma or ringworm received medical treatment, and were kept off the playgrounds until they had recovered.[497] Trachoma and ringworm, the two leading contagious diseases, were common among schoolchildren. The Hadassah Medical Organization's School Hygiene Department fought determinedly to overcome them, and enforced strict preventive rules. Children suffering from non-contagious diseases were treated at the playground by the nurse of the nearby school, who was also part of the staff. The nurse was responsible for medical supervision and for inculcating fundamental hygiene habits, such as cleanliness, proper use of toothbrushes and handkerchiefs, and hygiene in matters of food and clothing. Every day, children could be seen standing outside the playground fence, crying all afternoon, but refusing to go home and clean up. It can be said that this was the first time that these children had encountered a framework that demanded attention to personal hygiene as a condition for participation.

Jerusalem suffered from a water shortage, and this, of course, had a significant effect on the children's personal hygiene, and on the general state of hygiene and sanitation.[498] In mid-1928, at a time when houses did not yet have running water, the Har Zion B Playground was connected to the city water supply, and showers were installed. This could not be other than an attraction, and the children were wildly enthusiastic. Malka Koriel related that "there was no running water at home, and even the well-to-do families of the Ohel Moshe neighborhood did not have showers. Once a week, on Fridays, we came to the playground with soap and a towel and took showers, boys and girls, taking turns."[499]

However, the children's parents, and their Arab neighbors, strongly opposed the new practice. They considered collective bathing to be immoral, and refused to permit their sons and daughters to take a shower, lest they end up wandering naked in the streets. Only after it was explained to them that the children washed in an enclosed room — and that boys and girls washed separately — did they agree. The showers aroused amazement in the entire area, and attracted a never-ending flow of Arab visitors to the Har Zion B Playground to see the children come to shower in their free time and of their own free will, without having to either bring or pay for water.

Through these free hot showers, and strict adherence to rules of personal hygiene, the playground staff managed to indirectly instill these habits in the children's homes as well; parents also began to observe basic rules of cleanliness and hygiene. Thus, the playground became a powerful educational factor, instilling the foundations of health teachings throughout the entire community.

Epilogue

Three hundred children participated regularly in the activities held in the first playground opened in Eretz Israel in 1925. Within five years, the scope of the enterprise had tripled. By 1930, there were three playgrounds, two in Jerusalem (Har Zion B and Machane Yehuda) and one in Tel Aviv, which hosted in all 1,400 children. By 1947, there were 40 playgrounds across the country, attended by a total of 7,000 children. Activity ceased in most of the playgrounds during the Israel War of Independence in 1948, and as the State of Israel was established 24 of the playgrounds renewed their activities; their annual budget reached 20, 000 Eretz Israel pounds, and was funded by the Hadassah Youth Council.[500]

Along with the permanent playgrounds, seven temporary summer playgrounds were also opened in 1948, for a period of between two and four months. Between 2,000 and 2,500 children participated in activities there every day. A recreation camp was also established at Kfar Vitkin, which hosted 300–400 children every summer, in two-week sessions. The summer playgrounds were set up in urban areas or in villages and farms where permanent lots could not be obtained, for budgetary or technical reasons. The activities offered to the children in these playgrounds included sports, games, crafts, field trips, and camping, and they were directed by counselors who were for the most part teachers or students at teacher-training colleges or universities.

In 1935, the Central Youth Bureau was established, as a division of the Department of Education of the National Jewish Council in Eretz Israel, headed by Yosef Meyuhas.[501] Youth Bureau activities focused mainly on educating neglected teenagers in the slums and immigrant towns, and in cultivating informal Hebrew education. Its areas of responsibility included "...a) supervising the Guggenheimer-Hadassah playgrounds; b) supervising the youth clubs of the Jewish volunteer organizations in Eretz Israel; c) organizing courses for counselors for the above activities, which laid the foundation for training professional manpower for leading youth."[502]

In 1951, three years after the establishment of the State of Israel, the volunteer organizations were transferred to the State and the playgrounds were moved from Hadassah's auspices to those of the Ministry of Education. The Youth Bureau of the National Council became the Youth Department of the Ministry of Education and Culture, and the Ministry took over the budgeting and staffing of the playgrounds.

The singularity of the Guggenheimer-Hadassah playgrounds, in comparison to other playgrounds in the world, lay in their attempt to actualize political goals (Arab-Jewish) and to bridge cultural gaps (religious-secular), along with fulfilling educational goals and providing compulsory free medical services as part of the overall program to educate a new generation in Eretz Israel, healthy in body and spirit. Even though the success of these goals were limited and it did not create a new relationship between Arabs and Jews, the experience itself was unique and pioneering, leading to a greater understanding of the gaps between the two communities and that playing together was not enough to overcome them. But, from an educational point of view, it can be said that the playgroundsprogram was a great success and that it laid the infrastructure for the development of informal education in Eretz Israel and in the State of Israel.

Appendix
School Hygiene Department (1921)[503]

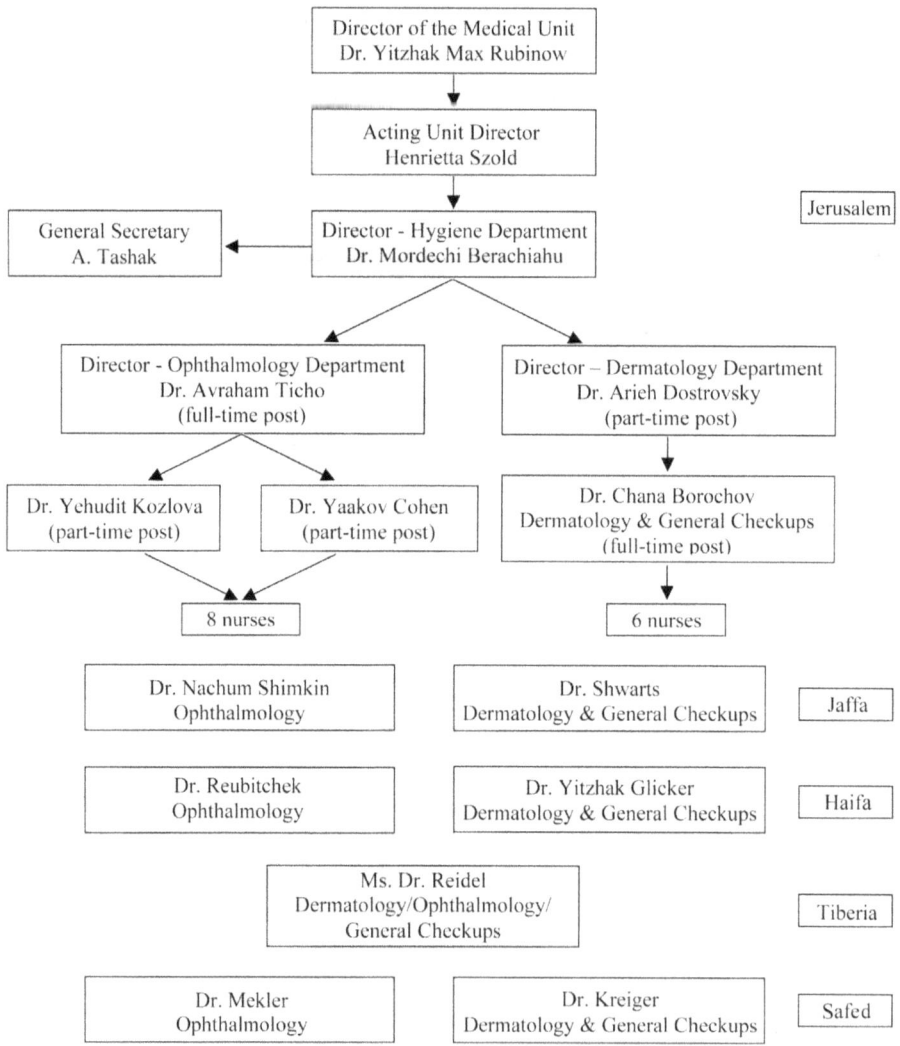

Director of the Medical Unit
Dr. Yitzhak Max Rubinow

Acting Unit Director
Henrietta Szold

Jerusalem

General Secretary
A. Tashak

Director - Hygiene Department
Dr. Mordechi Berachiahu

Director - Ophthalmology Department
Dr. Avraham Ticho
(full-time post)

Director – Dermatology Department
Dr. Arieh Dostrovsky
(part-time post)

Dr. Yehudit Kozlova
(part-time post)

Dr. Yaakov Cohen
(part-time post)

Dr. Chana Borochov
Dermatology & General Checkups
(full-time post)

8 nurses

6 nurses

Dr. Nachum Shimkin
Ophthalmology

Dr. Shwarts
Dermatology & General Checkups

Jaffa

Dr. Reubitchek
Ophthalmology

Dr. Yitzhak Glicker
Dermatology & General Checkups

Haifa

Ms. Dr. Reidel
Dermatology/Ophthalmology/
General Checkups

Tiberia

Dr. Mekler
Ophthalmology

Dr. Kreiger
Dermatology & General Checkups

Safed

The Structure of the School Hygiene Department

Personnel and Budget[504]

Department Budget	4,519 Eretz Israel pounds
Number of Pupils Supervised by the Department	25,000
Number of Educational Institutions Encompassed	270

Breakdown of Medical Staff	
Physician-Director	1
Full-time Physicians	2
Part-time Physicians	3
in Villages (Moshavot)	25
Chief Nurse-Executive Nurse	1
Public Nurses	14
Part-time Secretary (see chart)	1

Trachoma

Budget for the war on trachoma	5,424 Eretz Israel pounds
Number of pupils Infected with trachoma under the Department's supervision	2500
Number of families infected with trachoma under the Department's supervision[505]	1000

Medical Team	
Ophthalmologists	4
Traveling doctor[506]	1
Nurses	24
Secretary	1

The following data from five out of twenty schools in Jerusalem, reflects the scope of work:

Table 1

Percent of Patients with Ringworm Among Schoolchildren,
According to School Attended at Beginning (Before Treatment)
and End of the Year (After Treatment) 1920–1921[507]

School	Enroll-ment	No. with Ringworm At Beginning of the Year	No. with Ringworm At End of the Year	No Cured	Percent Cured
Boys' School	290	38	22	16	42.1%
Tachkomoni School	368	85	48	37	43.5%
Talmud Torah Sfardi	152	97	26	71	73.2%
Girls' School	542	120	75	45	37.5%
Kindergarten	114	17	12	6	29.4%

Table 2
Results of Treatment of Trachoma[508]

City	1919	1937	No. of Students
Jerusalem	21.6%	2.2%	14201
Tel Aviv	64.8%	4.4%	17345
Safed	55%	2.3%	530
Tiberias	78.3%	13.5%	1209
Villages	64-65%	3.2%	14924
Haifa	49%	3.75%	6617
		TOTAL: 3.65%	TOTAL: 4826

The Development of Playgrounds in Eretz Israel Source:
Annual Report of Hadassah-Guggenheimer
Activities for the year 1948/9 (CZA, J17/432).

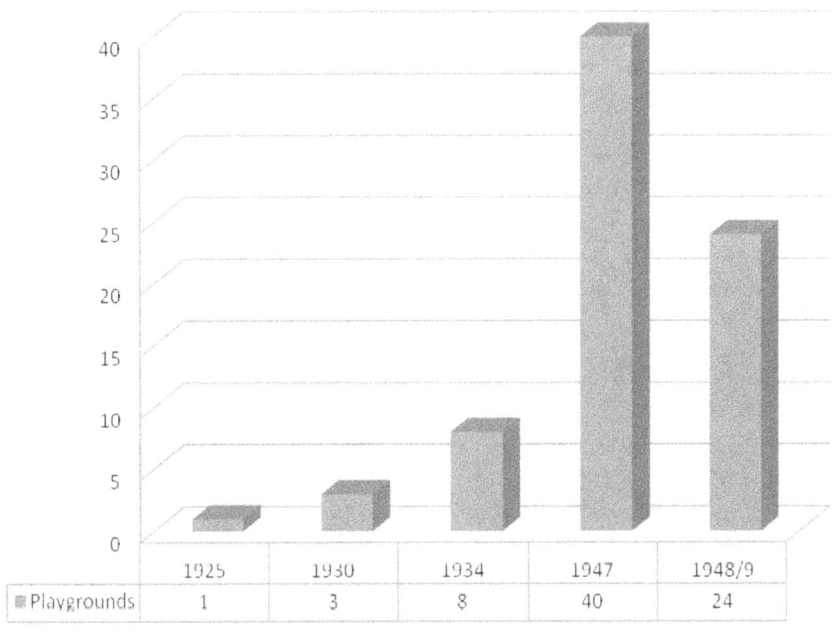

	1925	1930	1934	1947	1948/9
Playgrounds	1	3	8	40	24

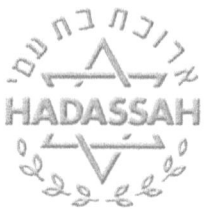

Notes

1. Richard Gottheil was the son of Rabbi Gustav Gottheil, who immigrated from Germany to the United States and became the rabbi of Temple Emanuel, a Reform congregation in New York. In 1897 he was elected president of the Zionist Executive (Hamerkaz Hatzioni) and was destined to later head the American Zionist Federation. U. J. Melvin, **American Zionism from Herzl to Holocaust**, New York, 1976 p. 80, On Gottheil and the influence of his leadership on the Zionist movement in the United States, A. Frizel "ha-Manchigut ba-Tnua ha-Zionit b-Artzot ha-Brit, 1900–1930" (Leadership in the Zionist Movement in the United States 1900–1930) in A. Malchi and Z. Tzachor (eds.). **Manhig u-Manhigut** (Leader and Leadership), Jerusalem, 1992, pp. 191-195.

2. On Emma Gottheil (1862–1947) and her Zionist activity, C. Kutscher-Bosworth. **The Early Years of Hadassah 1912–1921**, Ph.D. dissertation, Brandeis University, 1976, p. 100; Herzl encouraged the wives of Zionist leaders to take a part in activities of the Zionist movement, and said: "What are women for Zionism, I don't want to say: 'Nothing.' What can they do and what should they do, perhaps everything!" F. Yaffe, (Hebrew) "The Woman in the Zionist Congress," **Ha-Isha** (The Woman), 1917, p. 3.

3. Magnes (1877–1948) served as Reform rabbi at Temple Emanuel. In 1922 he immigrated to Israel and was among the leading proponents of Jewish-Arab cooperation — in favor of establishment of a bi-national Jewish-Arab State as a solution to the problem of Eretz Israel. In 1952 he was appointed the first rector of the Hebrew University in Jerusalem, and from 1937 until the day of his death served as president of the Hebrew University. Frizel (footnote 1) p. 192.

4. Constitution of Hadassah (CZA J113/1661).

5. On Henrietta Szold's first visit to Eretz Israel in 1909, M. Lowenthal, **Szold: Life and Letters**, New York, 1962, pp. 67-68.

6. On Eva Leon's philanthropic work on behalf of establishment of a nursing center in Israel, Kutscher-Bosworth (Footnote 2), p. 101.

7. D. Ben-Gurion, **Zichronot (**Memoirs), Vol. 3, Tel Aviv, 1987, p. 112.

8. A. Gal, "Medinat Yisrael ha-Idealit b-Einei Hadassah" (The Ideal State of Israel in the Eyes of Hadassah), 1945–1955," **Yahadut Zmaneinu**, 4 (1988), pp. 157-159. On the influence of American progressivism on the work of Henrietta Szold, M. Brown, "Henrietta Szold's Progressive American Vision of the Yishuv" in A. Gal (ed.) **Envisioning Israel**, Jerusalem 1996, pp. 62-80.

9. *"Is there no balm in Gilead? Is there no physician there? Why then is not the health of the daughter of my people recovered?* (Jeremiah 8:22)

10. M. Levin, **Benot Hayil Irgun Hadassah, 1912–1987** (Hadassah Women of Valor, 1912–1987), Tel Aviv, **1987**, p. 8.

11. D. Shapira, **Tahalichei Bniyah shel Moetzet ha-Chirum ha-Zionit k-Zeroa ha-Peulah ha-Tzionit Medinit shel ha-Zionut ha-Amerikayit 1938–1944** (The Process of Building the Zionist Emergency Council as an Arm of American Zionist Political Activity 1938–1944), Ph.D. thesis, Hebrew University, 1979, p. 189.

12. Ben-Gurion labeled Hadassah "the biggest organized power in America", Ben Gurion, **Zichronot** (Footnote 7), vol.3, p. 77; "This is the strongest federation in the city." In Y. Erez (ed.), **Igrot Ben-Gurion** (Ben-Gurion's Letters), Vol. 3, Tel Aviv 1971, p. 178.

13. **Ha-Isha**, 5 [2nd Year], 1928, p. 22.

14. Nathan Straus (1848–1931), Jewish philanthropist and owner of the department store chain Macy's in New York, was actively involved in health matters in his city and during the years 1893–1919 established and funded operation of a network of milk distribution stations for infants whose mothers could not nurse. His interest in Eretz Israel was aroused under the influence of Judah-Leib Magnes. In 1912, Straus began to take steps to improve health services among Jewish and Arab communities in Israel. G.A. Rosen, **A History of Public Health**, New York, 1976, p. 355; A Frizel, **Ha-Tnua ha-Zionit be-Artzot ha-Brit ba-Shanim 1897–1914** (The Zionist Movement in the United States Between the Years 1897–1914), Tel Aviv 1970, pp. 164-165.

15. A network of home nursing services was established in the United States in 1893 by Lilian Wald (1867–1940), a Jewish nurse born in Cincinnati, Ohio. During her work as a nurse in a New York hospital, Wald was exposed to the distress of immigrant women. Motivated by a desire to help them, she moved into their neighborhood on 265 Henry Street on the Lower East Side, opening the Nurses' Settlement House on the premises — a framework that provided home nursing services to the local population. In time, the house became a community center that led the way to organization of a permanent voluntary organization called the Visiting Nurse Service of New York City. L. D. Wald, **The House on Henry Street**, New York, 1915.

16. R. Makover, **Shilton u-Minhal be-Eretz Israel, 1917–1925** (Government and Administration in Eretz Israel, 1917–1925), Jerusalem, 1988, pp. 166-167.

17. Kupat Holim — whose full name in Hebrew is Kupat Holim Ha'Clalit or The General Sick Fund, but is referred to in this

volume simply as "Kupat Holim" —originally defined itself in 1911 as "the emissary of the organized working public in the Federation of Labor in matters of health in Israel." Its role was to extend medical assistance to its members, their families and parents; extend financial assistance to its members in times of illness; organize the workers' health matters; and serve as social-medical insurance for the working public in Israel. In 2010 Kupat Holim is still the major public health provider in Israel serving over 50% of the population. Shvarts, S., **The Workers' Health Fund in Eretz Israel,** NY and UK, 2002.

18. A. Boehm, **Ha-Milchama, ha-Briut veha-Machalot ha-Midabkot be-Eretz-Israel** (The War, Health and Contagious Diseases in Eretz Israel), Jerusalem 1915, pp. 8-14.

19. N. Levi, **Prakim be-Toldot Harcfua be-Eretz-Israel 1797–1948** (Chapters in the History of Medicine in Eretz Israel), Tel Aviv, Haifa 1998, pp. 170-174; Henrietta Szold said about the activity of the Red Cross that "the country having known war and known suffering was in need of a medical and nursing endeavor of larger dimensions than what the Red Cross could supply." The Red Cross left the country in 1919. Henrietta Szold, **Hadassah be-Eretz-Israel** (Hadassah in Eretz Israel) 1920–1929, a speech delivered at the festive opening of the Nathan and Lina Straus Health House in Jerusalem on April 30, 1929.

20. Ch. Sh. Halevi, "Hadassah, Histadrut Nashim Tzioniot b-America" (Hadassah), **Encyclopedia ha-Ivrit (**The Hebrew Encyclopedia), Vol. 13, Jerusalem and Tel Aviv 1969, p. 616.

21. **$356,000.00** in the year 2009 has the same "purchase power" as **$25,000** in the year 1918, Lawrence H. Officer and Samuel H. Williamson, "Purchasing Power of Money in the United States from 1774 to 2010," MeasuringWorth, 2009. URL http://www.measuringworth.com/ppowerus/result.php

22. **Hadassah Bulletin**, 33 (1917), p. 8.

23. At first, Dr. Y. S. Hirsch from New York was appointed director of the Unit, however during 1918 he announced that for personal

reasons he would not be able to depart for Eretz Israel, and Henrietta Szold sought a replacement. In order not to delay departure of the Unit, Dr. Benyamin Roman was appointed acting director until a permanent director could be found. Dr. Rubinow was appointed in the last quarter of the year, and his request that he be allowed to settle his affairs and join the Unit at a later date was accepted. D. H. Miller, **A History of Hadassah 1912–1935**, Ph.D. dissertation, New York University 1968, pp. 244-245.

24.   The American Association for Labor Legislation operates today as a research institute and archive under the auspices of Cornell University in New York, dedicated to documentation of activity for progressive legislation. R. Numbers, **Almost Persuaded**, Baltimore and London 1978.

25.   Shvarts S., and Brown T., "Kupat Holim, Dr. Isaac Max Rubinow and the American Zionist Medical Unit's Experiment to Establish Health Care Services in Palestine 1918–1923", **Bulletin of the History of Medicine**, 1998, 72(1)28-46.

26.   Dr. Rubinow, Personal Letters (AALL I-11-4); T. Brown, **Jewish Physicians in the USA**, Tel Aviv 1995, pp. 221-233.

27.   S. Shvarts, "Beit ha-Holim Sha'ar Zion – Beit ha-Holim ha-Kehilati ha-Rishon b-Aretz" (Sha'ar Zion Hospital – The First Community Hospital in Israel) in **Koroth**, 9 (9-10), 1989, pp. 292-308.

28.   J. L. Kreader, "Isaac Max Rubinow: Pioneering Specialist in Social Insurance" in **Social Service Review,** 9 (1976), pp. 405-411.

29.   In May 1921 marauding Arab mobs attacked Jews, first in Jaffa and adjacent Jewish neighborhoods in Tel Aviv, with violence then spreading to five Jewish agricultural towns in the coastal plain on the Tel Aviv periphery. The "1921 disturbances," as they were labeled, engineered to erupt as if in response to May Day demonstrations by Jewish workers, had been organized in advanced by extremist elements in the Arab camp opposed to Zionism and Jewish immigration. During the outburst, 95 persons were killed and 219 seriously injured — including Jewish author

Josef Haim Brenner who was murdered by Arab rioters in Jaffa. Walter Laqueur, **A History of Zionism**, London 1972 p. 209.

30. R.Mohilever-Zukerman, "Tziunei Deresh" (Milestones), **Ha-Achot** (The Nurse), 6 (January, 1947) p. 10.

31. In the last stages of the war, as the British front advanced, Turkish authorities deported the Jews of Tel Aviv to the interior of the country.

32. Z. Carmi, **Mechanekh Ve-Darco** (An Educator and His Way), Haifa, 1965, p. 211.

33. S. Shvarts, and T. Brow, "Kupat Holim, Dr. Isaac Max Rubinow and the American Zionist Medical Unit's Experiment to Establish Health Care Services in Palestine 1918–1923", **Bulletin of the History of Medicine**, 72(1), pp. 28-46, 1998.

34. D.Niederland, "Haspaat ha-Rofim ha-Olim me-Germania al ha-Histpatchut ha-Refuah b-Eretz-Israel 1933–1948" (The Influence of Immigrant Doctors from Germany on the Development of Medicine in Eretz Israel 1933–1948) **Cathedra**, 30 (December 1984), pp. 114-115.

35. Numbers (Footnote 24), pp. 16-17.

36. Szold speech (Footnote 19), pp. 5 6.

37. Rubinow's response to a letter published in the Hebrew daily *Haaretz*, protesting against "the regulation instigated by Hadassah, that physicians are not permitted to engage in private practice," **Ha-Aretz**, 15.7.1922; the Unit doctors' constitution and their salaries, and the decision approved in their meeting regarding denial of the right to private practice (CZA, J113/1366); memorandum from Dr. Rubinow regarding prohibition of engaging in private practice, 26.10.1924 (CZA, J113/1434).

38. Hadassah Medical Organization, Third Report, September 1920–December 1921. Jerusalem 1922, pp. 40-41; 49-56; 70-73.

39. Rubinow's Files. Notes from: September 10, 1919; March 1, 1920; August 13, 1920; February 13, 1921(AALL Series I, Box 111, File 4); Levontin to Szold, 5.11.1920 (Hadassah Archives, NY 7-10-111).

In this letter to Szold, Levontin relates to Rubinow's treatment of new immigrants, and Rubinow's aspirations to create a medical network similar to the American hygiene system that required every immigrant to undergo a medical examination at Ellis Island before entering the United States. The objectives were to make medical supervision possible, protect the local population from contagious diseases and instill in immigrants proper hygienic and nutritional habits.

40. Latvian-born Dr. Berachiahu (1882–1959), a member of the Second Aliyah, studied in Switzerland and served as school physician for the Herzliya Gymnasium in Tel Aviv between 1912 and 1919. During World War I he served as a military doctor in the Turkish Army. After the war, he was appointed director of the School Hygiene Department. D. Margalith, **Physicians Forerunners of Modern Israel**, Tel Aviv 1973, pp. 67, 69; N. Levi, **b-Sherut ha-Kihila, Hakibutz Hameuchad Pub. & Bnei Zion Medical Center, Haifa, 1997** (In the Service of the Community), p. 35.

41. H. Yaffe, **Dor Maapilim** (A Generation of Ascenders), Jerusalem 1975, pp. 539-565; Dr. Arieh Boehm, director of the Pasteur Institute in Jerusalem, "ha-Halacha le-Maaseh" (Realization), **Ha-Poel ha-Tzair**, 12 (13) 1919. (The article describes the demeaning attitude of Dr. Berachiahu and Unit physicians toward veteran local doctors.)

42. Hadassah Medical Organization (footnote 38), pp. 12-13.

43. Yaffe (footnote 41), p. 366.

44. "le-Shealat Sidur ha-Refua b-Eretz-Israel" (The Question of the Medical Setup in Eretz Israel), **Ha-Poel ha-Tzair**, 19 (13), 1919; Dr. I. M. Rubinow, "Avodat Hadasssah b-Eretz-Israel" (Hadassah's Work in Eretz Israel), **Ha-Aretz**, 25.7.1919; Takanot v-Hachlatot Kupat Holim (Regularions and Decisions Kupat Holim), Jaffa (1913) **Ha-Achdut**, Kislev TAR'AB (1912), p. 22.

45. Hadassah Medical Organization (38), pp. 12-13.

46. **Protocol ha-Veidah ha-Shniyah shel ha-Histadrut ha-Klalit shel ha-Ovdim ha-Ivriim b-Eretz-Israel** (Protocol

of the Second Convention of the General Federation of Labor of Hebrew Workers in Eretz Israel), Tel Aviv 1923, p. 25; D. Ben-Gurion, "ha-Poel ha-Ivri vha-Histradrut," **Tarbut ve-Chinuch**, Tel Aviv 1964, p. 122.

47. Z. Tzachor, **Shorshei ha-Politika ha-Yisraelit** (Roots of Israeli Politics), Tel Aviv 1987, pp. 34-35.

48. Miller (footnote 23).

49. Ibid., pp. 260-263.

50. Niederland (footnote 34), pp. 114-115.

51. D. Fox, **Health Policies**, New Jersey 1986, pp. 14, 82, 85.

52. **Pinkas**, Jerusalem 1923 (supplement) Kupat Holim-Hadassah (Sick Fund-Hadassah), chapter 10-11, pp. 15-17.

53. Miller (Footnote 23), pp. 131-141.

54. Heskem Kupat Holim-Hadassah (Sick Fund-Hadassah Agreement), October 1922 (LA IV 243-1).

55. **Pinkas** 7 (Footnote 52).

56. Parting words of Dr. Rubinow at the party held in his honor by Hadassah women upon his departure in 1922 (AALL 11-4).

57. Rosen (footnote 14), pp. 365-382.

58. Dr. Alexandra Belkind (1871–1943) was the first school physician at Herzliya Gymnasium. She received her medical training in Paris and afterwards specialized in gynecology and pediatrics in Geneva. In 1904 she opened a private clinic in Jaffa, offering gynecological treatment. In 1908 she began working in Herzliya Gymnasium, She continued to practice medicine in Tel Aviv until the end of her life. A. Weitzbard, "Masechet ha-Rofim ha-Rishonim b-Rishon le-Tzion" (A Chapter in the First Doctors in Rishon le-Zion) **Koroth**, 6 (11-12) 1975, pp. 738-756.

59. Mordechi Karishovski-Ezrachi (1862–1951) immigrated to Eretz Israel from the Ukraine in 1887. For six years he served as a Hebrew teacher in the Alliance School in Jerusalem. In 1894, he was appointed principal of the Hovavei Zion Girls' School

in Jaffa. He was among the leading figures in the Teachers' Federation. His work to advance the training of teachers using Hebrew as the language of instruction was realized by the Ezrah Society that established a teaching seminary (1904), the first of its kind in Eretz Israel. M. Rinot, **Chevrat ha-Ezrah le-Yehudei Germania b-Yetizirah ub-Maavak** (The Ezra Society for German Jews in Work and Struggle), Jerusalem 1972, pp. 109-110, 239.

60.   This visit constituted a turning point in the Zionist activity of Henrietta Szold. M. Urofsky, **American Zionism from Herzl to Holocaust**, New York 1976, p. 132; Lowenthal (footnote 5), pp. 67-68.

61.   Y. Press, **Meah Shanah b-Yerushalayim (Hundred Years in Jerusalem)**, Jerusalem 1964, pp. 9-10.

62.   Czechoslovakia-born Dr. Avraham (Albert) Ticho (1883–1960) received a Jewish and general education. He studied medicine in Vienna and specialized in ophthalmological diseases and was a leading figure in the fight against trachoma in the schools and Talmud Torahs in Jerusalem. Between the years 1919 and 1921 he directed Hadassah Hospital's Ophthalmology Department. D. Tidhar, **Encyclopedia le-Halutzei ha-Yishuv u-Bonav** (Encyclopedia of the Yishuv's Pioneers and Builders), 2, Tel Aviv 1947, p. 956.

63.   The Education Committee was established during World War I by the Eretz Israel Office (representative of the World Zionist Organization within Eretz Israel). The Committee directed Hebrew schools supported by the Zionist movement and supervised Zionist-inspired schools in general.

64.   Y. Reuveni, **Mimshal Mandatori b-Eretz-Israel** (Mandatory Administration in Eretz Israel), Ramat Gan 1993, p. 180; D. Niederland, "Hashpaat Rofim Olim mi-Germania al Hitpatchut ha-Refua b-Eretz-Israel 1933–1948" (Influence of Immigrant Doctors from Germany on the Development of Medicine in Eretz Israel 1933–1948), **Cathedra**, 30 (December 1984), p. 114.

65. Ibid. pp. 188-189; Correspondence of Colonel Heron with the General Sick Fund (LA, IV 208-270B).

66. Jerusalem-born Dr. Rafael Oplatka (1884), studied medicine in Belgium and Beirut and worked for the Turkish government in the war against epidemics. In July 1920 with the organization of British civil government in the country, he continued his post as a doctor in the Government Health Department. In 1926, he was appointed chief physician and director of the Government Health Office in Tel Aviv, concentrating heavily on introduction of sanitary and hygienic facilities in educational institutions. Tidhar (footnote 62), B, p. 629.

67. Berachiahu to the head management of the Hadassah Medical Federation, 8.2.1929 (CZA J113/343); Letter reminder from Berachiahu to the head management of the Hadassah Medical Federation, 22.3.1932 (CZA J113/346).

68. Ibid., A.

69. Ibid.

70. Ibid.

71. Dr. Chaim Yasski, born in Kishinev in 1896, studied medicine in Odessa and Geneva, immigrated to Eretz Israel in 1920 and served as a Hadassah ophthalmologist in Haifa. Dr. Yasski headed the war to eradicate trachoma in the agricultural townships (*moshavot*) as a traveling doctor, later serving as director of the Ophthalmology Department at Hadassah Hospital in Jerusalem. From 1928, Dr. Yasski served as director of the Hadassah Medical Center. He was murdered on April 13, 1948, near Sheik Jarach on the outskirts of Jerusalem — one of 78 medical personnel in the convoy of doctors and nurses on their way to the Hadassah Hospital complex on Mount Scopus, attacked by Palestinian Arab insurgents. Tidhar (footnote 62), 4, p. 1770; Margalith (footnote 40), p. 75.

72. Berachiahu (footnote 67), A.

73. Ibid., B.

74. Berachiahu to the Education Department, Zionist Executive, 15.10.1929 (CZA J113/344).

75. Ibid.

76. Dr. Reuven Katzenelson, born in Russia in 1890, completed his university studies in Napoli with a doctorate in political and social science. In 1914 he immigrated to Eretz Israel. Between the years 1922 and 1930 Dr. Katzenelson served as deputy administrative director of Hadassah. In 1931, he was appointed director of the Popular Sick Fund (*Kupat Holim Amamit*) established by Hadassah. Tidhar (footnote 62), pp.305-306.

77. Yasski to Katzenelson, 5.7.1929 (CZA J113/343). See also: The same to Szold, 12.2.1930 (CZA J113/344).

78. Ibid.

79. Professor Israel-Yaakov Kligler was born in the Ukraine in 1889, and immigrated to the United States in 1901. He completed his Ph.D. in Biology, Bacteriology and Public Health at Columbia University in New York. In 1921 he immigrated to Eretz Israel as a member of the American Zionist Medical Unit, and began working as head of the Unit's Bacteriology Lab in Hadassah in Jerusalem. In 1923, he established and headed the Malaria Research Institute — the first facility to engage in preventive medicine in the country. Professor Kligler also directed the Straus Health Center in Jerusalem. establishing the pasteurization of milk and distribution of milk to schools services. Tz. Saliternik **Korot ha-Milchama b-kadachat v-Eretz-Israel v-Hadbarata** (Regarding the War of Malaria in Eretz Israel and Its Eradication), Jerusalem, 1979, p. 75.

80. Protocol "ha-Vaada le-Cheker Darkei Peulah shel Machleket ha-Higiyena" (Protocols of the Committee for Investigation of Operative Avenues for the Hygiene Department), 3.1.1932 (CZA, J113/346).

81. Ibid.

82. Ibid.

83. Yasski to Berachiahu, 12.1.1932 (CZA, J113/346).

84. A daily payment of an industrial worker was about 30 mils. Dan Giladi, Jewish Palestine During the Fourth Alia Period, 1924–1929, Am Oved, Tarbut Vechinuch, Tel Aviv 1973, TASHLAG pp. 83-84.

85. Yasski to Levi, Alliance School in Jerusalem, 5.4.1922 (CZA, J113/341).

86. The Education Department was established by the Zionist Commission (*Va'ad Hatzirim*) at the end of the First World War. From a budgetary standpoint, the Education Department was the largest among the Departments (Aliyah or Immigration Department, Settlement Department, etc.) established by the Zionist Commission. The Department was under the authority of the Education Committee. R. Elboim-Dror, **Ha-Chinuch Ivri b-Eretz-Israel** (Hebrew Education in Eretz Israel), 2, Jerusalem, 1990, pp. 3, 36; Y. Berkson, **Machleket ha-Chinuch shel ha-Hanhalah ha-Tzionit b-Eretz-Israel, Sidura v-Hanhalata** (The Education Department of the Zionist Executive in Eretz Israel, Its Order and Administration), Jerusalem 1929, pp. 13-19; Y. Bentowitz, **Ha-Chinuch b-Medinat Yisrael** (Education in the State of Israel), Tel Aviv 1960, p. 31.

87. Ibid.

88. Ibid., p. 30.

89. In Hebrew: Zerem Haovdim, a small number of special elitist schools designed for the children of labor leaders and close associates.

90. On the problems of dividing schools into three educational/political streams: The main General stream, the Workers' (i.e. Socialist) stream and the Mizrachi (i.e., religious) stream, and aspirations to unite all Hebrew education under the management of the Zionist Federation, Berkson Tz. Tzameret, "Esser Shnot Chinuch" (Ten Years of Education), Tz. Tzemeret and Ch. Yablonka (eds.), **Ha-Asor ha-Rishon** (The First Decade — 1948–1958), Idan, 20, Jerusalem 1997, pp. 125-127.

91. Berachiahu to Hadassah management, 18.5.1931 (CZA, J113/345).

92. Berachiahu to Head Management of Hadassah, 22.8.1928 (CZA, J113/342).

93. Ibid.

94. Protocol of a meeting of the Hygiene Committee associated with the School Hygiene Department, 19.2.1922 (CZA, J113/341).

95. Berachiahu to Hadassah management, 13.9.1935 (CZA, J113/348).

96. Ibid.

97. Protocol "ha-Vaada le-Cheker Darkei Peulah shel Machleket ha-Higiyena" (Protocols of the Committee for Investigation of Operative Avenues for the Hygiene Department), 3.1.1932 (CZA, J113/346).

98. Ibid.

99. Berachiahu to Hadassah Management, 13.9.1935 (CZA, J113/348).

100. Ibid.

101. Ibid.

102. Berachiahu to Henrietta Szold, 1931. (CZA, J113/345).

103. Berachiahu to Hadassah management, 13.9.1935 (CZA, J113/348).

104. Berachiahu to Hadassah management, 13.10.1935 (CZA, J113/348).

105. Berachiahu to Hadassah management, 15.11.1935 (CZA, J113/348).

106. Yasski to Berachiahu, December 1931 (CZA, J113/345).

107. Protocol "ha-Vaada le-Cheker Darkei Peulah shel Machleket ha-Higiyena"[Protokol of the Hygiene Department](footnote 97).

108. Berachiahu to Berkson, director of the Education Department, Jewish Agency, 11.1.1932 (CZA 113/346).

109. Berachiahu to Head Management of Hadassah, 18.5.1931 (CZA, J113/345).

110. Joint meeting of delegates from Hadassah, Kupat Holim and Culture Committee of the Labor Federation "on the subject of finding medical assistance for schools within the network of the Culture Committee of the Labor Federation." 6.2.1923 (CZA J113/341).

111. Berachiahu to Hadassah management, 27.3.1931 (CZA, J113/345).

112. Berachiahu to Hadassah management, 18.5.1931 (CZA, J113/345).

113. Berachiahu to Hadassah management, 21.2.1935 (CZA, J113/348).

114. Summary of a discussion on hygiene matters at schools, 14.3.1935 (CZA J113/348).

115. Minutes from the first meeting of the professional committee for preventive work 12.6.1935 (CZA, J113/348).

116. Berachiahu to Katzenelson, 17.4.1923 (CZA J113/434).

117. Berachiahu to Hadassah management, 6.1.1929 (CZA, J113/475).

118. Berachiahu, reminder to Hadassah management: "Avodat Machleket ha-Higiyena shel Beit ha-Sefer" (Work of the School Hygiene Department), 27.3.1931 (CZA J113/345).

119. The Second School Physicians' Convention, **Ha-Aretz**, daily newspaper, 26.3.1928; The decisions of the second school physicians' convention, CZA J113/342.

120. Berachiahu to architect Fritz (Peretz) Kornburg, 17.1.1928 (CZA, J113/342).

121. Announcement from Bluestone, 18.3.1928 (CZA, J113/342).

122. B. Tamir, "Ha-Achot Bertha Landsman," **Ha-Achot**, 3, p. 9-12; On the appointment of Bertha Landsman, the Hebrew newspaper, **Davar**, 9.7.1925.

123. Bluestone to Berachiahu, 9.11.1928 (CZA, J113/342).

124. This is a clear innuendo regarding the foreign origins of Bertha Landsman, who in the estimation of Berachiahu sought to apply an American work system in Eretz Israel. Berachiahu always stressed that one should create a hygiene culture according to

prevailing conditions of the People and the land of Eretz Israel and not to "copy everything from other countries, but to set a special plan of action according to conditions in our country and the goals to which we aspire in our Return to our homeland." Berachiahu, The school and the Pupil in Eretz Israel, Jerusalem, 1928, p. 5.

125. Berachiahu to Hadassah management, 21.2.1928 (CZA J113/342). Emphasis in the original.

126. Ibid.

127. Bertha Landsman to Yasski, Re: Proposals for Re-Organization of Hygiene Nursing Schools, 10.4.1932 (CZA J113/346).

128. Yasski to Berachiahu, 27.5.1933 (CZA J113/346).

129. Z. Brunn, **Sidur ha-Milchama neged ha-Gar'enet** (Arrangements for the War against Trachoma), Jerusalem, 1916, p. 3.

130. Berachiahu to Hadassah management, 9.7.1928 (CZA J113/342).

131. "She'elon b-Nogea le-Batei-Kissei v-Haspakat ha-Mayim b-Batei ha-Sefer b-Moshavot — Machleket ha-Higiyena" (Questionnaire Regarding Toilets and Water Supply in Schools in the Agricultural Townships — Hygiene Department), (Undated), (CZA J113/342).

132. Borodetzky to Berachiahu, 17.11.1924 (CZA J113/476).

133. Borodetzky to Berachiahu, 15.12.1924 (CZA J113/476).

134. Borodetzky to Berachiahu, 17.1.1925 (CZA J113/477).

135. Berachiahu to Levontin, director of the Jaffa branch of Hadassah, 27.7.1924 (CZA J113/476). Emphasis in the original.

136. Berachiahu to Hadassah management, 18.11.1927 (CZA J113/342).

137. Ibid.; "An Overview of the Work of the Hadassah Medical Federation." A lecture given by Dr. Bluestone, Hadassah director, in a press conference organized by the Keren Hayasod or Foundation Fund — the financial arm of the World Zionist Movement, 9.6.1925 (LA Unit IV 243/1222).

138. Meeting of school physicians, Tel Aviv September 1923 (CZA J113/341).

139. Ibid.

140. Berachiahu, Pupils' Clinic, October 1927 (CZA J113/342).

141. Ibid.

142. A radioisotope used by physicians to treat ringworm.

143. Dr. Arieh Dostrovsky, born in Russia in 1887, studied medicine at the universities of Vienna and Basel, specializing in dermatology and venereal diseases. In 1919 he immigrated to Eretz Israel and began working as head of the Department of Dermatology and Venereal Diseases in Hadassah Hospital, until the opening of the Hebrew University Hospital on Mount Scopus (1939). He was appointed the first dean of the medical school of the University and Hadassah during the years 1949–1950. Dr. Dostrovsky served as chairman of the Union of Dermatologists in Eretz Israel. Tidhar(footnote 62) vol. IV, p. 1749.

144. Ibid.

145. At this time, there were no microscopes in Palestine or knowledge of how to use them. Malaria was diagnosed by clinical symptoms of the disease and by an enlarged spleen. Tz. Saliternik, **Korot ha-Milchama b-Kadachat b-Eretz-Israel v-Hadbarata** (Regarding the War on Malaria in Eretz Israel and Its Eradication), Jerusalem 1979, p.21.

146. Berachiahu, "Avodat ha-Hegiena b-Betei ha-Sefer" (Hygiene Work in the Schools), **Sefer ha-Yovel shel Histadrut ha-Morim** 1903–1928 (Jubilee Book of the Teachers' Federation), 1, Jerusalem 1929.

147. Ibid., p. 284.

148. "Chagigat ha-Machzor ha-7 le-Beit ha-Sefer le-Achayot Hadassah b-Yerushalayim" (Seventh Graduating Class Celebration of the Hadassah Nursing School in Jerusalem), **Ha-Isha** [The Women], 1 (2nd Year) 1927, p. 30.

149. The "Health Fellowships" were established in 1928 among students in the upper classes who were chosen to help the school nurse in her work, to instill good hygiene habits and maintain cleanliness of school premises. R. Guchmann, "Agudot ha-Briut b-Betei ha-Sefer ha-Amami'im b-Aretz" [The Health Fellowships in Elementary Schools in Eretz Israel], **Ha-Achot** [The Nurse], 4 (1943), pp. 26-41. Z. Shehory-Rubin, "Health Leagues, Health Scouts and Health Week: 'Hadassah's Tools of Propaganda for the Promotion of Health in Eretz Israel during Mandatory Times", **Korot** 17 (2003-2004), pp. 31-46. (Hebrew)

150. Berachiahu, Jubilee Book (footnote 146), p. 284.

151. Berachiahu to Hadassah management, 30.4.1923 (CZA J113/475). For comparison, it should be noted that school physicians at the time received a monthly salary of 16 Eretz Israel pounds.

152. Berachiahu to Hadassah management, 17.4.1931 (CZA J113/345).

153. Berachiahu Ibid.

154. Berachiahu to Hadassah management, 24.3.1926 (CZA J113/201).

155. Protocol of a meeting of doctors and nurses, 17.6.1929 (CZA, J113/343).

156. Protocol of the annual meeting of nurses in preventive services in Eretz Israel, **Haachot**, [The Nurse], IV, 1943.

157. An annual countrywide "Health Week" was organized jointly by the Hygiene Department, the Straus Health House in Jerusalem and Tel Aviv, the Labor Federation Sick Fund and the Health Committee of Knesset Israel — **the latter a representative body of Jewish inhabitants of Eretz Israel during the British Mandate.** The week was devoted to discussions, lectures and activities on the subject of health and was planned by pupils and their families. The protocol of a meeting of the advisory committee associated with the Department for Public Health Education, Nathan and Lina Straus Health House, Jerusalem, 11.5.1932 (CZA, J113/1445). See also **Health Week in Palestine** (CZA J113/1445).

158. Y. Press, **Eleh Toldot Beit ha-Sefer leha-Atzil le-Beit Lamel b-Yerushalim** (And This is the History of the Nobel House of Lamel School in Jerusalem), Jerusalem 1936, p. 10.

159. Ibid., p. 13.

160. Rinot (footnote 59) p. 106.

161. Elboim-Dror, (footnote 86), p. 21.

162. A. Hacohen-Avidor, **Ha-Ish Neged ha-Zerem** (The Man Against the Stream), Jerusalem 1975, pp. 81-82.

163. Berachiahu (footnote 146) p. 37.

164. Ch. Sh. Halevi, records clerk to Dr. Yitzhak Alterman, director of the Education and Culture Department of the Tel Aviv Municipality, 16.4.1936 (CZA J113/498); Dr. Borodetzky, physician responsible for school hygiene work in Tel Aviv, memorandum on treatment of skeletal defects, 18.6.1936 (CZA J113/498).

165. Berachiahu (Footnote 146), p.37.

166. Report by Dr. Berachiahu to Hadassah management 30.3.1925 (CZA J113/477).

167. Berachiahu to Hadassah management, 20.3.1923 (CZA, J113/475).

168. Berachiahu (footnote 146), p. 38.

169. **Protokol ha-Veida ha-Shnia shel Rofei Batei ha-Sefer** (Protocol of the 2nd Convention of School Physicians), 1.4.1928 (CZA J113/342).

170. Ibid.

171. Berachiahu to Dr. Eliezer Reiger, 6.3l.1929 (CZA J113/342).

172. Berachiahu to Hadassah management, 29.11.1928 (CZA J113/342).

173. Ibid. It should be noted that already in 1741 a French doctor by the name of Nicolas Andry warned of many defects and physical deformities among children stemming from deficient treatment in childhood. In his opinion one of the means of preventing

skeletal defects was adjustment of chair size to the age and height of the children. Therefore, he designed a special chair for children that could be adjusted according to the height of the child and sitting position. Nicolas Andry, **Orthopaedia: or The Art of Correcting and Preventing Deformities in Children**, Philadelphia and Montreal 1961, pp. 82-85.

174. Berachiahu to Professor Kligler, 18.5.1932 (CZA J113/346).

175. Berachiahu to Yitzhak Alterman, director of the Education and Culture Department of the Tel Aviv Municipality, 15.6.1936 (CZA, J113/498).

176. Ibid.

177. Ibid., p. 128.

178. Elboim-Dror (footnote 86), B, p. 346.

179. Berachiahu, circular to school principals, 8.2.1928 (CZA, J113/342).

180. Ibid.

181. Ibid.

182. Berachiahu, **Nohalim le-Yetiziah le-Tiyulim** (Procedures for Going Out on Hikes), 11.3.1931 (CZA, J113/345).

183. **Protokol ha-Veida ha-Shnia shel Rofei Batei ha-Sefer** (Protocol of the 2nd Convention of School Physicians), 1.4.1928, (CZA J113/342).

184. T. Grushka (ed.) **Health Services in Israel**, Jerusalem 1968, p. 59.

185. A. Dostrovsky, "ha-Milchama b-Machalot Or ha-Midabkot" (The War on Contagious Skin Diseases), **Ha-Chinuch**, 9, 1926, p. 98; **Op. Cit** "Histpatchut ha-Dermatologia b-Eretz-Israel," **Harefuah**, 47, Pamphlet 12, (December 1954), pp. 252-253.

186. M. Berachiahu, **The school and the Pupil in Eretz Israel**, Jerusalem, 1928, p. 17.

187. Berachiahu to Hadassah management, 22.8.1942 (CZA J1113/342).

188. Ibid.

189. Ch. Yasski, **Mah Yesh le-Daat le-Briut ha-Einayim?** (What's Important to Know about Eye Health?), Jerusalem 1927, p. 1 (Physicians' House Archive — Menachemia).

190. H. Yaffe, **Ha-Milchama Neged ha-Garenet b-Ezrat Chofshim v-Ozrim Refui'im Nimuchim** (The War Against Trachoma with the Aid of Paramedics and Low-Level Medical Aids), Jerusalem 1915, p. 7, (Physicians' House Archive — Menachamia).

191. Z. Brunn, **Sidur ha-Milchama Neged ha-Garenet** (Organization of the War Against Trachoma), Jerusalem 1915, p. 8 (Physicians' House Archive — Menachamia).

192. D.M. Karinkin, **Ha-Garenet b-Eretz-Israel al pi Praksisei ha-Prati** (Trachoma in Eretz-Israel in my Private Practice), Jerusalem 1915, p. 1. (Physicians' House Archive — Menachamia).

193. Yasski (footnote 189), p. 1.

194. D.M. Karinkin, "ha-Garenet b-Batei ha-Sefer ha-ivri'im b-Eretz-Israel v-Emtzaei ha-Milchana b-machalah Zot" (Trachoma in the Hebrew Schools in Eretz-Israel and Means of Fighting this Disease) **Ha-Chinuch**, 1 (1914) pp. 21-56; M. Shimkin, "Hamilchama b-Garenet" (The War on Trachoma), **Ha-Chinuch**, 8 (1925), pp. 31-39; Grushka (footnote 184), pp. 59, 108.

195. Physicians' House Archive — Menachamia. Emphasis in the original.

196. Karinkin (footnote 192), p. 47.

197. Y. Kozlova, "Nisayon le-Kidum (Prophlaxis) Dalakot Midabkot shel Einayim" (Experience in Advancing Prophylaxis of Contagious Eye Inflammations), **Harefuah**, 4, Pamphlet 5 (1927), pp. 251-254.

198. Berachiahu to Hadassah management, 22.12.1926 (Hadassah Archives — New York, 7/11/119C).

199. Ibid. Dr. Feigenbaum also suggested "to offer small prizes to children who exhibit perseverance in receiving eye treatment." Feigenbaum to Bluestone, 5.12.1926 (Op. Cit.).

200. Kozlova to Yasski — Hadassah management, 5.6.1929 (CZA, J113/346).

201. Kozlova to Yasski — Hadassah management, 13.3.1932 (CZA, J13/346).

202. Feigenbaum to Berachiahu, 3.8.1930 (CZA, J113/344).

203. Ibid.

204. Yasski to the Education Department, 7.8.1930 (CZA J113/344).

205. Berachiahu to Szold, 19.12.19211 (CZA, J113/341).

206. Ibid.

207. Ibid.

208. Berachiahu to the Sanitation Committee of the Tel Aviv Municipality, 7.12.1925 (CZA, J113/478). Emphasis in the original.

209. Berachiahu, "Chozer l-Kol Achayot Batei ha-Sefer" (Circular to All School Nurses), 23.2.1932 (CZA J113/346).

210. Berachiahu to the Education Department, 13.8.1931 (CZA, J113/345).

211. Ibid.

212. Berachiahu to Dr. Yosef Luria, director of the Education Department, 8.11.19831 (CZA, J113/345).

213. Berachiahu to the Education Department, 11.2.1924, (CZA, J113/476).

214. Borodetzky to Berachiahu, Summer 1926 (CZA, J113/342).

215. Berachiahu to architect Mr. Kornburg, 17.1.1928 (CZA, J113/342).

216. Berachiahu to the branch of the Society of Engineers and Architects in Eretz Israel, to Chairman A. Kook, Jerusalem, 5.3.1928 (CZA, J113/342).

217. **Protokol ha-Veida ha-Shnia shel Rofei Batei ha-Sefer** (Protocol of the 2nd Convention of School Physicians), 1.4.1928 (CZA J113/342).

218. Berachiahu to the Education Department, 20.1.1930 (CZA 113/344).

219. Ibid.

220. Ibid.

221. Dr. Berachiahu to the Education Department, 30.1.1930 (CZA J113/344).

222. Ibid.

223. Dr. Berachiahu to the Education Department, Report on the visit of Dr. Mirenburg, 18.11.1930 (CZA J113/344).

224. **Pratei Kol Asefat Achiyot b-Yerushalaim** (Protocol of a Nurses' Meeting in Jerusalem), 1.5.1931 (CZA J113/345).

225. **Pratei Kol Asefat Achiyot b-Yerushalaim** (Protocol of a Nurses' Meeting in Jerusalem), 29.5.1931 (CZA J113/345).

226. Ibid.

227. Berkson to Berachiahu, 27.5.1932 (CZA J113/347). For comparison purposes it should be noted that in the same year (1932), a school nurse received a salary of 7 Eretz Israel pounds and a school physician 16 Eretz Israel pounds.

228. Berachiahu to Berkson, 28.5.1932 (CZA, J113/347).

229. Ibid.

230. Protocol of **Ha-Vaada l-Cheker Darkei Peula shel Machleket ha-Higiena** (Committee for Investigation of Avenues for Action of the School Hygiene Department), 3.1.1932 (CZA J113/346).

231. Gringer, to Alterman, 18.2.1936 (CZA J113/498).

232. Patterns of Immigration to Eretz Israel since the establishment of the Zionist movement have come in mass waves of immigration (*Aliyah* in Hebrew) — the most recent being that of Russian Jews in the early 1990s. Those waves prior to the establishment of the

State of Israel in 1948 are numbered — the wave that brought Jews primarily from Germany being termed the Fifth Aliyah. D. Niederland, "Hashpaat ha-Rofim ha-Olim mi-Germania al Hitpatchut ha-Refuah b-Eretz-Israel, 1933–1948" (The Influence of Immigrant Physicians from Germany on the Development of Medicine in Eretz Israel, 1933–1948), **Cathedra**, 30 (December, 1984), pp. 118, 124.

233. Ibid., pp. 127-135, Y. Gelber, **Moledet Chadasha** (New Homeland), Jerusalem, 1990, pp. 344-414; Y. Reuveni, **Mimshal ha-Mandat b-Eretz-Yisrael** (The Mandatory Government in Eretz Israel), Ramat Gan, 1993, p. 186.

234. The Ezrat Nashim Society that was organized in Jerusalem in 1890, with the goal of providing support for ill women and indigent new mothers, established a hospital in 1895 for the mentally ill. Levi (footnote 19), p. 82.

235. German-born Dr. Chaim (Heintz) Hermann, (1892–1948), received his medical education in Germany specializing in neurological diseases and mental illness. In 1924 he immigrated to Eretz Israel where he practiced neurology and psychiatry. Dr. Hermann directed the hospital for the mentally ill, *Ezrat Nashim*, in Jerusalem, and served as chairman of the Neurological-Psychiatric Society in the country. He was a lecturer on mental illness at the Hadassah-run Nursing School and was appointed as a legal expert on questions of mental illness by the British Mandatory government. D. Tidhar (footnote 62) p. 1922.

236. Gelber (footnote 233), p. 443.

237. Within the medical and educational field, it is customary to classify retarded children into three groupings: 1. Untrainables with an IQ up to 25, who are totally disconnected from the outside world; 2. Trainables with an IQ up to 50, who can be trained and taught to a limited extent; 3. Educables with an IQ of 50-75 who can be trained and educated. Tz. Shtall, "ha-Yeled ha-Zakuk l-Chinuch Miyuchad" (The Child in Need of Special Education), Y. Nir (ed.), **Pirkei Chinuch Meyuchad** (Chapters in Special Education), Jerusalem 1970, (1975) pp. 44-46.

238. Berachiahu to Szold, 7.11.1932 (CZA, J113/347).

239. The Ben Shemen and Meier Shfeyah youth villages were agricultural-educational institutions that accepted orphaned children and the sons of Zionist families in the Diaspora in order to give them an education in Eretz Israel. The goal was to found their education upon training to establish new agricultural settlements in Eretz Israel, opening the door to a new, healthier life. Agricultural youth villages were part of a broader Zionist agenda for the return of Jews to their homeland imbued with aspirations for a revolution in patterns of Jewish life in the Diaspora that included a return to the soil and nurturing a Jewish farmer class. The first and most outstanding institutions of this kind were the Mikve Israel School (1870), the Meier Shfeyah Youth Village (1904) and the Ben Shemen Youth Village (1927). Ch. Rinot, "ha-Chinuch ha-Pnimiati b-Chevah Mishtanah" (Boarding School Education in a Changing Society), V. Ackermann, A, Carmon, D. Tzuker (ed.), **Ha-Chinuch b-Chevrah Mithavah** (Education in a Nascent Society), 2, Tel Aviv and Jerusalem 1985, p. 722; Y. Bentvitz, **Ha-Chinuch be-Medinat Yisrael** (Education in the State of Israel), Tel Aviv 1960, pp. 256-257.

240. Berachiahu (footnote 238).

241. Sh. Zaks, "Al K'shaei Chinuch k-Etgar la-Mechanech" (On Learning Disabilities as a Challenge for Educators), Y. Nir. (ed.) **Pirkei Chinuch Meyuchad** (Chapters in Special Education), Jerusalem 1975, pp. 27-37.

242. The Consultation Stations operated according to the Heal-Pedagogic method. This approach was developed in Europe in the 1930s, founded by H. Hanselman who defined it as "an educational doctrine and concern for all children whose physical and psychological development has been impaired over a long period by social and individual factors, including children with impaired senses, children with slow development and children with *a neurotic*_constitution." According to this doctrine, the child is first examined by a physician. If it is found that he needs mental care, it is given by an educator who is specially

trained for this role, under the supervision of a doctor. N. El-Ad, A Wiener, **Sherut ha-Mivchan le-Noar v-Toldot ha-Tipul be-Yeladim ub-Nearim Azuvim v-Ovrei Chok** (Probation Services for Youth and the History of Treatment of Abandoned Children and Delinquents), Tel Aviv 1995, p. 163.

243. Berachiahu, "Hegeina Ruchanit b-Mosdot ha-Chinuch" (Mental Hygiene in Educational Institutions), **Higiena Ruchanit** (Mental Hygiene) 10, 36 (1947), p. 27.

244. Berachiahu, **Beit ha-Sefer veha-Talmid b-Eretz-Israel** (The School and the Pupil in Eretz Israel), Jerusalem (1938) p. 22.

245. Berachiahu to Berkson, director of the Education Department, 25.6.1930 (CZA J113/344).

246. Memorandum written by Berachiahu, 26.9.1932 (CZA J113/347).

247. Romanian-born Dr. Elchanan Rabinowitz (1896–1957), received his M.D. from the University of Vienna. He immigrated to Israel in 1919 and began working at Hadassah Hospital in Jerusalem. In time he became the director of the Pediatrics Department, chairman of the Medical Federation in Jerusalem and chairman of the Pediatricians' Federation N. Levi, Y. Levi, **Rofaia Shel Eretz Israel** (The Physicians of the Holy Land) 1799-1948, Zichron Ya'akov, 2008, p. 341.

248. Protocol of a meeting, 23.3.1930 (CZA J113/344).

249. Ibid.

250. Ibid.

251. Berachiahu to Hadassah management, 16.5.1932 (CZA J113/346).

252. Ibid.

253. Berachiahu to Hadassah management, 1.6.1930 (CZA J113/345).

254. Berachiahu (footnote 243), p. 42.

255. It has been a matter of long-standing tradition — prompted by the Zionist ethos of "a return to the soil" — for public schools in Israel to expose all schoolchildren to agricultural life through maintenance of garden plots.

256. It is important to cite that despite the huge achievement inherent in the establishment of the first school for retarded children, the school constituted a marginal solution relative to the large number of retarded children in the country. In Tel Aviv alone there were at this time over 600 children with mental retardation. Berachiahu to Alterman, 22.3.1936 (CZA, J113/347).

257. Grumann in a memorandum regarding a school for retarded children, 15.9.1935 (CZA J113/498).

258. Grumann in a memorandum and report on the institution for retarded children, 29.1.1936 (CZA J113/498).

259. Berachiahu to Hadassah management, 16.5.1932 (CZA J113/346).

260. During the years 1918–1922 there was only one type of educational-social institution in Germany and Austria — the reformatory. The first reformatory was established in Eretz Israel for juvenile delinquents along the same lines. D. Reifen, **Ha-Katin u-Beit ha-Mishpat l-Noar** (The Juvenile and Juvenile Courts), Tel Aviv, 1978, p. 42; A Eichorn, **Noar Azuv** (Abandoned Youth), Jerusalem 1972, p. 121.

261. Protocol of a meeting of the committee assigned the question of child criminals, 14.6.1932 (CZA J113/347); in article 18 (6) of the Juvenile Offenders Ordinance of 1937 there was a directive that the scout could order whipping a young offender as punishment. Whipping as a punishment, more than any other punishment, carried a strong element of humiliation that had no correlation to punishment or rehabilitation of the young offender. The article was abolished by Israeli lawmakers at the end of British Mandate rule, who stressed "There will be no whipping as punishment in the State [of Israel]." (Law Abolishing Whipping as a Punishment — 1950)` Y. Horowitz, "le-Sheelat ha-Makot l-Avaryanim Ze'irim" **Yediot al ha-Avodah ha-Sotzialit b-Aretz** (News on Social Work in Israel), 8 (1936), p. 183-185.

262. Protocol of a meeting of the committee (footnote 261).

263. The "Big Brother" program matched non-professional adult males to young delinquents who met on a regular weekly basis

so that the former would exert a positive influence through their character, direct interest and material assistance rendered to the latter. N. El'ad and A Wiener, **Sherut ha-Mivchan le-Noar v-Toldot ha-Tipul be-Yeladim ub-Nearim Azuvim v-Ovrei Chok** (Probation Services for Youth and the History of Treatment of Abandoned Children and Delinquents), Tel Aviv, 1995, p. 163., p. 78.

264. The first playgrounds were established in the United States at the end of the eighteenth century and were intended to prevent delinquency and to serve as an educational tool for youth and development of character. This was one of the goals of playgrounds established in the mid 1920s in Eretz Israel by Hadassah. Z. Shory-Rubin and S. Shvarts, The Guggenheimer-Hadassah Playgrounds in the 1920s, **Cathedra**, 1998(86) pp. 75-98.

265. Szold to Berachiahu, 11.5.1933 (CZA, J113/347).

266. Berachiahu, A Survey on the Institutions for Juvenile Delinquents in Tul Karem, 21.6.1933 (CZA J113/364).

267. Protocol of the committee, 28.6.1932 (CZA J113/364); (CZA A419/96).

268. Ibid.

269. Szold to Berachiahu, 20.4.1933 (CZA, J113/364); With a fund donated by the Jewish philanthropist Kaduri, an agricultural school for Arab youth was established in Tul Karem, to parallel the Kaduri Agricultural School in the Jewish settlement of Kfar Tabor in the Galilee. Reuveini, **Memshal ha-Mandat** (Mandatory Government), p. 164.

270. Szold to the Governing Committee of Meir Shfeyah, via Dr. Berkson, 9.9.1932, (CZA, J113/347).

271. Ibid.

272. Ibid.

273. Szold to Berachiahu, 21.9.1932 (CZA, J113/364).

274. Berachiahu to Szold, 23.9.1932 (CZA J113/364).

275. Ibid.

276. Ibid.

277. Ibid.

278. Berachiahu to Szold, 21.11.1932 (CZA J113/347).

279. Berkson to Szold, 3.11.1932 (CZA J113/347).

280. Szold to Berachiahu, 3.11.1932 (CZA J113/347).

281. Berachiahu (footnote 243), p. 42.

282. Shehory-Rubin Z., Shvarts S., "The Guggenheimer- Hadassah playgrounds in Jerusalem", **Cathedra,** 86:75-98, 1998 and in Shehory-Rubin Z and Shvarts S.,"Teaching the Children How to Play – The Establishment of the First Playgrounds in Palestine during the British Mandate Period" **Israel Studies**, 15 (2) (2010), pp. 24-48. See also chapter V.

283. G. Finn, **Eitot Sufa** (Seasons of Storm), Jerusalem, 1980, pp. 330, 332.

284. M. Montefiore, **Moshe ve-Yerushalayim** (Moshe and Jerusalem), translated by David Garrdan, 1866, pp. 10-11.

285. M. Eliav, **Be-Chasut Mamlechet Austria 1849-1917** (Under Imperial Austrian Protection 1849–1917), Jerusalem, 1986.

286. Ibid., pp. 98-99.

287. Ibid., pp.101-102.

288. Ibid., pp. 101-102; B. Tz. Gat, **Ha-Yishuv ha-Yehudi be-Eretz Israel be-Shnot 1940-1881**, (The Jewish Yeshuv in Eretz Israel in the Years 1881–1940) Jerusalem, 1974, p. 149.

289. N. Levi, **Perakim be Toldot Ha-Refuah** (Chapters in the History of Medicine), pp. 125-126; Shmuel Nissan and Petra Martin, "Das Marienstift-Kinderhospital (1871-1899)" in **Historia Hospitalium,** Zeitschrift der Deutschen Gesellschaft fur Jerusalem, Krankenhausgeschichte, Heft 20 (1995-1997), pp. 162-188. The hospital building is located on Hanevi'im Street 29. Upon the initiative of Professor Shmuel Nissan, the Jerusalem Municipality placed a plaque marking the building.

290. **Din ve-Cheshbon Shnati shel ha-Histadrut Nashim Ivriot**, (Annual Report of the Hebrew Women's Federation), Jerusalem Branch 1925.

291. Eliyahu Parush, one of the first officials at the Sha'arei Tzedek Hospital wrote that in the Gynecology Department "older women and beside them several girls who had learned the craft" worked "because then there were not young experts as nurses. A registered nurse was brought from Holland to teach the profession to girls." A. Parush, **Sha'arei Tzedek: le-Toldot Beit ha-Holim Sha'arei Tzedek ve-Yerushalim ve-Rofavu oo-Menahalo ha-Rishon ha-Doktor Moshe Wallach** (Sha'arei Tzedek: The History of the Sha'arei Tzedek Hospital in Jerusalem, Its Physicians and First Director Dr. Moshe Wallach), Jerusalem, 1952, p. 29.

292. **Z. Shehory-Rubin,** "'And God was favorable to the midwives': Jewish midwives in Eretz Israel during the late Ottoman Period", **Massekhet**, 8 (October 2008), pp. 51-95.

293. A. Yellin, **le-Tzeetza'ai** (To My Offspring), Jerusalem 1941, p. 34; H. Kagan, **Reshit Darkai le-Yerushalayim** (My First Steps in Jerusalem), Jerusalem, no date cited, p. 36.

294. Ibid., p. 52.

295. Ibid.; In the mid–eighteenth century the method of tightly binding infants was still widely employed throughout Europe, including immobilizing the newborn's hands and feet based on the belief that the child could not maintain its body straight unless bound in diapers and strips of bunting. Beginning in the eighteenth century and into the nineteenth century, physicians in Western Europe fought this method and considered it groundless. In England and France mothers went over to the method of less restricted and light diapering, but in Germany doctors continued to fight tight swaddling of infants into the mid–nineteenth century — a method that remained entrenched in Eastern and Southeastern Europe until the mid–twentieth century. A. Stah "Hitpatchut Minhad Chitul ha-Tinukot be-Edot Shonot oobe-Meuchad etzel ha-Yehudim: Skirat Mekorot"

(Development of Diapering Customs of Infants Among Various Ethnic Groups Particularly Among Jews: Survey of Sources), **Korot,** 8 (1983), pp. 247-251.

296. Ay. Schmelz, "Kavim Meyuchadim be-Demographia shel Yehudei Yerushaliyim ve-Meah ha-19" (Special Patterns in the Demography of Jews in Jerusalem in the Nineteenth Century) in M. Eliav (ed.) **Prakim be-Toldot ha-Yishuv ha-Yehudi be-Yerushalayim** (Chapters in the History of the Jewish Yishuv in Jerusalem), Jerusalem, 1976, p. 545.

297. Ch. Sh. Halevi, **Chakirot be-Tmutat ha-Tinukot ha-Yehudi'im ba-Aretz** (A Study of Infant Mortality Among Jews in the Land of Israel), Jerusalem, 1941.

298. Helena Kagan (1889–1978), born in Tashkent, graduate of medicine in Bern, Switzerland, immigrated to Israel at the beginning of 1914 at the age of 25. She was to become one of the pioneers in pediatrics and among the outstanding personalities in Eretz Israel medicine. Z. Shehory-Rubin, "Dr. Helena Kagan (1889-1978): The First Paediatrician in Israel", **Journal of Medical Biography**, 16 (3) (August 2008). pp. 144-149.

299. Kagan (footnote 293), p. 45.

300. B. Gruenfelder, "Neged Mikrei ha-Mavet bein Tinukot be-Eretz Israel" (Against Mortality among Infants in Eretz Israel), **Ha-Poel ha-Tzair**, No. 28-29 (1914), pp. 19-21; as above "ha-Gorem ha-Sotziali be-Tipul ha-Tinokot" (The Social Factor in Care of Infants), **Yidiot al ha-Avodah ha-Sotzialit be-Eretz Israel** (Information on Social Work in Eretz Israel), 9-10 (July 1937), pp. 163-164.

301. B. Gruenfelder, "Infant Mortality in Palestine," **The Jewish Social Service Quarterly**, Vol. IX, No. 3 (June 1933), p. 309.

302. B. Gruenfelder, "Hitpatchut ha-Tipul be-Yonkim oobe-Olelim be-Shloshim ha-Shanim ha-Achronot" (Development of Care of Nursing Infants and Babies in the Past 30 Years), **Harefuah**, 29, Pamphlet 1, 1945.

303. **Din ve-Cheshbon Shnati shel Histadrut Nashim Ivriot** (Annual Report of the Hebrew Women's Federation) 1925.

304. Ibid.

305. Bat-Sheva Kesselman was a member of Hadassah before she immigrated to Eretz Israel. Upon her arrival in 1919, she encountered harsh realities — precarious conditions in which women gave birth and terrible infant morality rates. Aware of the power of organization, she formulated the idea of organizing groups of local women to cooperate with Hadassah in reaching out to expectant women and infants to offer assistance. Ay. Greenberg, Ch. Herzog **Irgun Nashim Volentari be-Chevrah Mithava** (Volunteer Women's Organization in an Emerging Society) Tel Aviv 1978, p. 14.

306. **Takanot shel Histadrut Nashim Ivriot** (Charter of the Hebrew Women's Federation), Jerusalem 1920.

307. Ibid.; "ha-Veidah ha-Shnatit shel Hey. Nun. Aleph. be-Eretz Israel" (The Annual Convention of the H.W.F. in Eretz Israel), **Ha-Isha**, 4, Second Year (1928), p. 26.

308. Veidat Histadrut Nashim Iviriot (Convention of the Hebrew Women's Federation), 23-24.3.1924 (CZA J35/7).

309. B. Gruenfelder, "Emunot-Shav ve-Minhagim Tfeilim be-Tipul be-Yonkim oobe-Gil ha-Yankut (False Beliefs and Unsavory Customs in Care of Nursing Babies and during Infancy), **Ha-Isha**, 3 (1928), pp. 23-26.

310. "Beit ha-|Tinukot" (The Infant House), **Ha-Isha**, 8 (1927), p. 33.

311. "Va'ad ha-Ganim" (The Kindergarten Committee), **Ha-Isha**, 8 (1927), p. 22.

312. Rubinow to Szold, 1921 (CZA J113/1346).

313. Ibid.

314. Rubinow, 15.6.1921 (CZA J113/1345).

315. Szold to Berlin, deputy chairperson of the Hebrew Women's Federation, 17.11.1922 (CZA J113/1346).

316. Rubinow to Szold, 12.5.1921 (CZA J113/1346).

317. B. Tamir, "he-Achot Berta Landsman (le-Yoflah ha-Shishim)" (Nurse Bertha Landsman [on her 60th Birthday]), **Ha-Achot**, 3 (1942), p. 9.

318. Ibid.

319. Ibid.

320. Ibid.; B. Landsman, **Infant Welfare Work Done by Hadassah Medical Organization in Jerusalem,** written in July 1923 for H.M.O. Report to XIII Congress Carlsbad in August 1923, (Hadassah Archive, New York RG/72/1).

321. Nissenbaum to Szold, 15.9.1921 (CZA J113/1385).

322. L. Kleinman, "Gvulot ha-Avodah shel he-Achot ha-Tziborit veha-Ovedet ha-Sotzialit" (Limitations in the Work of the Nurse and the Social Worker), **Ha-Achot** 1943, p. 63.

323. Ibid.

324. Ibid.; Gruenfelder (footnote 309), pp. 23-26.

325. **A Review of Infant Welfare and Prenatal Work in Palestine, 1921–1926,** Hadassah Archive — New York RG/72/2.

326. Bertha Landsman to Henrietta Szold, 9.5.1922 (CZA J113/1385).

327. **Yishifva le-Sedur Avodah be-Shtei Tachanot ha-Yonkim** (Meeting for Arranging Work Schedule at Two Stations for Nursing Babies) (CZA J113/1385).

328. **Infant Welfare and Milk Distribution Work in Palestine,** 1923, Hadassah Archive — New York RG/72/1.

329. **Tizkoret al Merkaz ha-Briut "Hadassah" be-Sha'ar Shkhem Yerushalayim** (Memorandum on the Hadassah Health Center at the Nebulas Gate Jerusalem) 29.11.1926 (CZA J113/1390).

330. Landsman to Kagan, chairperson of the Hebrew Women's Federation; **Hanidon: Ezrat Ovdot Mitnadvot be-Tachanot ha-Tipul be-Yonkim** (Re: Assistance of Volunteer Workers

in the Stations for Care of Nursing Babies), 2.7.1925 (CZA J113/1346).

331. The term "sanitation physician" referred to doctors who engaged in environmental medicine, or as it is sometimes called, environmental health and sanitation. Testing of milk was one of the tasks of the sanitation physician in those days, as was monitoring the quality of pasteurized milk, as preserving its nutritional value also served as a convenient growth medium for pathogens. Availability of high-quality pasteurized milk was one of the main factors in reduction of infant mortality from intestinal ailments.

332. "The Milk Problem before the League," **Palestine Weeky**, October 30, 1925.

333. **Agreement between H.M.H. and the Tipat Chalav Committee**, 22.5.1925 (CZA J113/1346).

334. Ibid.; "ha-Avodah ha-Meshutefet shel Hadassah ve-Histadruth ha-Nashim ha-Ivriot ba-Aretz" (Cooperation between Hadassah and the Hebrew Women's Federation in the Land [of Israel]), **Ha-Isha**, 2, 2nd Year (1927), p. 29.

335. **Tizkoret shel Shtei Yeshivot shel Vaadat ha-Mirkaz le-Horaa** (Memorandum on Two Meetings of the Center for Instruction Convention), 17.9.1935, 25.9.1935 (CZA J113/1390).

336. Landsman to Goldman, nurse in the Haifa Mother & Child Health Center, 16.3.1927 (CZA J113/1400).

337. From survey given by Dr. A. M. Bluestone, Hadassah director, in a press conference organized by *Keren Hayasod* (Foundation Fund), the financial arm of the World Zionist Movement. 9.6.1927 (LA IV 243/1222).

338. Ay. Cohen, "ha-Tipul be-Nashim Harot U-be-Tinokot be-Eretz Israel al yadei Hadassah" (Care of Pregnant Women and Infants in Eretz Israel by Hadassah) **Ha-Isha**, 1 (Nissan 1926), p. 14; Bertha Landsman, **A Review of Infant Welfare and Prenatal Work in Palestine through 1921-1926**, Hadassah Archives — New York (RG72/1).

339. Szold to Katinka, chairperson of the Hebrew Women's Federation in Haifa, 8.12.1922 (CZA J113/1397).

340. Katinka to Szold, 20.12.1922 (CZA J113/1397).

341. Le Comite Francais de puericulture et Goutte de lait pour Haifa, A Jewish Women's Organization in Paris.

342. Katinka to Szold, 23.12.1923 (CZA J113/1397). Emphasis in the original.

343. Dr. Nachum Shimkin, Hadassah branch director in Haifa to the head management of Hadassah Medical Federation Jerusalem, 2.12.1923 (CZA J113/1397); **Infant Welfare and Milk Distribution Work in Palestine**, Hadassah Archive — New York (RG72/1).

344. Ibid.; N. Levi **be-Sherut ha-Kehilah** (In the Service of Society), Tel Aviv 1997, p. 38.

345. Delegate of the French Committee in Haifa Mrs. P. Segal to Haifa Women's Federation and Hadassah Medical Federation, via Mrs. Ladijinsky, secretary. 8.7.1925 (CZA J113/1398); **Davar** Hebrew daily, 5.10.1925, an announcement to its readers of cessation of support of the nursing baby station in Haifa by the French Committee. It should be noted that Hadassah was not interested in the interference of the French Committee in management of the Haifa Health Center, fearing loss of control by Hadassah. In one case, Hadassah turned down an offer from a Jewish women's organization in Strasbourg to fund, establish and run a Mother & Child Health Center in Jerusalem. Hadassah agreed to the plan but refused to allow the women to manage the station on their own. The proposal fell. Szold to Rosenthal-Bauman, Strasbourg 17.5.1922 (CZA J113/1385).

346. Landsman to Nissenbaum, Hadassah director in Haifa, 30.10.1928 (CZA J113/1401).

347. Protocol of a Nurses' meeting at the Public Health Station in Haifa, 16.6.1930 (CZA J113/1402).

348. Dr. Z. Avigdori, acting branch director of Hadassah in Haifa, to Hadassah management, 28.12.1927 (CZA 113/1400).

349. Yasski to Glicker, Kupat Holim in Haifa, 27.1.1930 (CZA 1113/1401).

350. Yasski and Katznelson to Gruenfelder, 12.5.1929 (CZA J113/1401).

351. Perlson, to Hadassah in Jerusalem, 15.7.1930 (CZA J113/1402). **In Hebrew, the term Tachanat Yonkim — Station for Nursing Babies -- is simple and concise.**

352. Nissenbaum to Hadassah management, 14.1.1930 (CZA J113/1401).

353. Yasski, to Glicker, Kupat Holim Haifa, 27.1.1930, (CZA J113/1401).

354. Yasski, to Kupat Holim Central Committee Tel Aviv, 8.6.1930 (CZA J113/1401).

355. Agreement reached at a meeting regarding the station for nursing babies, convened in the offices of Kupat Holim in Haifa, 28.11.1935 (CZA J113/1403).

356. Known for its large and powerful socialistic community, Haifa was called by the Israeli public "Red Haifa."

357. Health Centers in Tiberias (CZA J113/1391).

358. Report by nurse Rachel Pesach on work at the station for nursing babies in Tiberias, 1925 (CZA J113/1391).

359. Ibid.

360. Landsman to Goldman, Tiberias, public nurse, 11.6.1928 (CZA J113./1392).

361. Yasski, to Szold, 20.6.1929 (CZA J113/1392).

362. Landsman to Hadassah management Jerusalem, 5.9.1927 (CZA J113/1392).

363. February 1923–January 1924 Report written by R. Shapira, chairperson, Hebrew Women's Federation Safed, 20.1.1924 (CZA J113/1394).

364. Szold to Hebrew Women's Federation Safed, via President Z. Goldberg, 27.12.1923 (CZA J113/1394).

365. Szold to Hebrew Women's Federation Safed, January 1924 (CZA J113/1394).

366. Bromberg, to the director of Hadassah branch management Safed, 28.6.1931 (CZA J113/1395).

367. Landsman to nurse Friedman, 23.1.1930 (CZA J113/1395).

368. The Arab riots of 1929 — following a pattern similar to riots in 1921, but more wide-spread — erupted over the right to Jewish access at the Western Wall spreading throughout the country, including Safed, but were actually designed to spark British limitations on Jewish immigration to Eretz Israel. The toll of violence: 133 Jews were killed and over 300 seriously injured and widespread damage incurred to Jewish assets. Atlas Carta le-Toldot Eretz Israel (Carta Atlas of Eretz Israel), Carta Jerusalem 1974, Vol. 2, Map 79.

369. Report — Health Welfare of Safed, October 1931–3, written by nurse Chedva Hilfer (CZA J113/1396).

370. Ibid.

371. Ibid.; Two substitutes for breast milk existed at the time, when a mother's own milk production was insufficient or impaired by illness: cow's and goat's. Cow's milk was recommended as it was rich in protein, calcium and vitamin B and differences from breast milk were slight. Y. K. Gugenheim, **T'zunat ha-Adam** (Human Nutrition), Jerusalem 1976, p. 253; Kagan recommended cow's milk, citing the drawbacks of goat's milk: Infants, most of Middle Eastern origin, gained weight when fed goat's milk, but they were weaker and paler, suffering from severe anemia. With advances in biochemistry it was found that the cause of anemia cited by Kagan was lack of vitamin B12 — the reason the children were found to be susceptible to disease and more vulnerable in their first years of life. Kagan (footnote 293), p. 49.

372. Greenberg and Herzog (footnote 305) pp. 18-27; Ch. Tahon, "Likrat Veidat WIZO Ha Baa" (Toward the Coming Conference of Zionist Women), **Ha-Isha**, 2, 2nd Year (1927), pp. 6-8; "ha-Masa oo-Matan bein Histadrut Nasim Irvirot oovein Histadrut Olamit

le-Nashim Tzioniot" (Negotiation between the Hebrew Women's Federation and the World Federation of Zionist Women), **Ha-Isha**, 8 (1927), pp. 32-33.

373. Shenkar, in the name of Kupat Holim to Hadassah management Jerusalem, 5.9.1926 (CZA J113/1404).

374. Gruenfelder, to the Hadassah Medical Federation, via Dr. Yasski, 27.4.1930 (CZA J113/1405).

375. Ibid.

376. Protocol of a joint meeting of delegates of Hadassah and WIZO, 3.12.1933 (CZA J113/1407).

377. Protocol between delegates of Hadassah and WIZO, 15.2.1933 (CZA J113/1407); protocol of a meeting (that took place in the presence of the chairperson of World WIZO, Vera Weizman), 22.2.1933, ibid.; protocol of meeting, 20.4.1933, ibid.

378. **Tochnit le-Ichud Ha Tipul be-Yeladim be-Tel Aviv** (Plan to Unite Care of Children in Tel Aviv (CZA J113/1407).

379. Ibid.

380. Agreement from a meeting of the 15th governing committee of the Labor Federation, 24.12.1934 (CZA J113/1408).

381. Ibid.

382. Memorandum on meeting of the Labor Federation with Kupat Holim, 24.2.1934 (CZA J113/1408).

383. Rokach to Yasski, 7.6.1935 (CZA J113/1409); T. Ledijinsky (chairperson of the Department for Childcare, 1946–1951). **Yediot WIZO be-Yisrael**, 37 (August 1951), p. 28.

384. The need to open two additional Health Centers stemmed from rapid population growth beginning in 1933 — a year that constituted a turning point in the life of Tel Aviv. The Fifth Aliyah — the fifth wave of Zionist immigration to Eretz Israel —brought 30,000 newcomers in one year, and 42,000 in 1934, mostly German Jews spurred to uproot and immigrate to Eretz

Israel by Hitler's rise to power. Some 60,000 chose to settle in Tel Aviv. At the beginning of 1933, the Tel Aviv population stood at 50,000 inhabitants; by 1935 it had swelled to 120,000. G. Biger, "Hitpatchut ha-Shetach ha-Banui shel Tel Aviv ba-Shanim 1909–1934" (Development of Built-up Areas of Tel Aviv in the Years 1909–1934) in M. Naor (ed.) **Tel Aviv be-Reshita, 1909-1934**, Idan, 3, Jerusalem 1984, p. 60.

385. Yasski to Dizengoff, 13.3.1936 (CZA J113/1409).

386. Katznelson, 14.4.1936 (CZA J113/1409).

387. Ibid.

388. Ch. Sh. Halevi (ed.), **Esrim Snot Sherut Refui be-Eretz Israel, 1918-1936** (Twenty Years of Medical Service in Eretz Israel), Jerusalem 1939, p. 24.

389. **Tipul be-Yonkim** (Care of Nursing Infants), Hebrew Women's Federation, Jerusalem (CZA J113/1394).

390. Nursing is the recommended form of feeding for an infant during the first year of life. The advantages and importance in the physical and emotional development of the child much has been written about, beginning with Jewish sources. Sh. Kotek, "ha-Ha'anaka be-Mekorot ha-Yahadut — Historia ve-Halacha" (Nursing in Jewish Sources — History and Jewish Law), **Assia**, 7, (1980), pp. 45-53; Y. Guggenhaim, **Tzunat ha-Adam** (Human Nutrition), Jerusalem 1976, pp. 253-155.

391. Protocol of a meeting of nurses in charge of Health Centers in Jerusalem, 28.6.1935 (CZA J113/1390).

392. Landsman to Berachiahu, 17.10.1934 (CZA J113/1406).

393. **Tipul be-Yonkim** (footnote 389).

394. Ibid.

395. From a lecture delivered by Nurse Leah Gershonson to mothers at the Health Center in Haifa, 20.5.1933 (CZA J113/1399).

396. Zelda Goldman and Tzipora Ashkenai-Azulai, public nurses, "al Chagigat ha-Prasim shel Tachanot ha-Refuah ha-Tziburit be-

Haifa" (On the Prize-[giving] Celebration at Public Health Centers in Haifa), 25.5.2925 (CZA J113/1399).

397. Ibid.

398. "Chagiga ba-Tachana le-Tipul ba-Tinbokot shel Hadassah" (Celebration at the Hadassah Infant Care Station) **Ha-Isha**, 8 (1927) pp. 39-40.

399. Goldman and Ashkenai-Azulai (footnote 396).

400. Chagiga ba-Tachana (footnote 398).

401. A. Levine, secretary of the Education Department in Safed to Chaya Katzelnik, 23.7.1933 (CZA J113/1396).

402. Bertha Landsman, **Palestine Mothers and Babies Celebrate**, 10.4.1930 (CZA J113/1392).

403. Goldman and Ashkenai-Azulai (footnote 396).

404. Ibid.

405. Dr. Arieli, **Doch shel ha-Tachanah le-Tipul ba-Yonkim be-Yerushaliyim** (Report of the Station for Care of Nursing Babies in Jerusalem), 1934.

406. Dr. Katzenelson, deputy director of Hadassah, ordered establishment of a *Tipat Chalav* Fund in 1929, with the objective of collecting donations for "distribution of milk to infants in need." Money collected by the Fund was made available to the Hebrew Women's Federation in order to buy and distribute milk to infants in need in Jerusalem. The Women's Federation donated the sum of 5–10 Eretz Israel pounds per month on its own to this project. Dr. Katzenelson to the Financial Department, 12.9.1929 (CZA J113/15/5).

407. **Horaot bishvil ha-Machlevot: Klalim le-Shmirat ha-Nikiyon ba-Machlevot ha-Misapkot Halav le-Tipat Chalav: Nikui ha-Parah, Niju Harefet, Klei ha-Chalivah, Kadei he-Halav, Laboush HaCholev.** (Instructions for Dairies: Rules for Maintaining Cleanliness in Dairies Supplying Milk to *Tipat Chalav*: Cleanliness of the Cow, the Dairy, Milking

Equipment, Milk Cans and Attire for the Dairyman). Bertha Landesman to Zelda Goldman, public health nurse in Haifa, Rachel Cohen, delegate of the Women's Federation in Haifa, and Dr. Shimkin, Haifa branch director of Hadassah (CZA J113/1398).

408. Landsman to Zaslavsky, Hadassah Tel Aviv, 12.11.1931 (CZA J113/1405).

409. Landsman to Goldman, Hadassah Haifa, 12.11.1931 (CZA J113/1402).

410. Nurse R. Feldman, **Skirah shel Chagigat Yaldei-Maavar be-Tachana A b-Ir ha-Atika** (Survey of the Children-in-Passage Celebration at Station A in the Old City).

411. Leah Kleinman, Supervisory Nurse in Jerusalem, **Skirah al Chagigat Gmar Gil-Maavar be-Tachanot be-Yerushalayim** (Survey of Completion Ceremonies for Passage-Age [Children] in Stations in Jerusalem) 21.3.1935 (CZA J113/1390).

412. Nurse A. Karniel, **Tazkir al Chagigoat Yaldei Maavar be-Tachanah C, Beit Yaakov** (Memorandum on the Children-in-Passage Celebration at Station C, Beit Yaakov), Jerusalem 5.9.1935 (CZA J113/1390).

413. Dr. Ostrovsky, **Chagigat Gil Maavar be-Haifa** (The Passage-Age [Children] Celebration in Haifa), 24.4.1232 (CZA J113/1403).

414. Neighborhood elder Yaakov Hadas, who participated in celebrations at celebrations at Station C in the Beit Yaakov neighborhood of Jerusalem.

415. Zelda Goldman, protocol from a meeting of public nurses in Haifa, 21.3.1930 (CZA J113/1402).

416. Landsman to Glicker, Kupat Holim Haifa, 15.4.1928 (CZA J113/1401).

417. Gruenfelder to Yasski, 23.7.1930 (CZA J113/1402).

418. Protocol of a nurses meeting in Haifa 12.11.1934 (CZA J113/1389).

419. C. Yasski, "al Bea'iyot Achadot shel ha-Refua ha-Mona'at" (On a Number of Problems of Preventive Medicine) in **Yediot al ha-**

Avodah ha-Sotzialit be-Eretz Yisrael (News on Social Work in Eretz Israel) 3-4 (3rd year) Tevet-Shvat 1938, p. 85.

420. Landsman to Goldman, supervisory nurse, Hadassah Haifa, 20.3.1931 (CZA J113/1402).

421. B. Ostrovsky, "Toldot Machleket ha-Yeladim be-Beit Cholim Rothschild be-Haifa 1929-1957" (The History of the Pediatrics Department in Rothschild Hospital in Haifa 1929-1957), **Koroth**, 10 (1993-1994), p. 22.

422. Rachel Pesach, **Doch al P'eilutah shel ha-Tachana le-Tipul ba-Yonkim be-Tveria** (Report on the Activity of the Care for Nursing Babies Station in Tiberias) 1925 (CZA J113/1391).

423. Hedva Hilfer, **Rishimot he-Achot me-Tachanot Briut Petach Tikva, likrat Anaf ha-Avodah ha-Atidi "Rishimot Tikun Nefesh Ha-Em"** (Notes From the Nurse at the Petach Tikva Health Station Regarding Work in the Future "Rectifying the Mother's Soul") 24.12.1934 (CZA J113/1403).

424. Pesach to Landsman, 29.8.1930 (CZA J113/1388).

425. Tova Blecher, Protocol of a meeting of nurses responsible for Health Centers in Jerusalem, 4.10.1935 (CZAJ113/1390).

426. Pesach to Landsman, 29.8.1930 (CZA J113/1388).

427. Pesach and Kleinman to Landsman 31.7.1930 (CZA J113/1388).

428. Landsman to Yasski, 9.10.1930 (CZXA J113/1388).

429. Yasski to Rabbi Kook, Head of the Rabbis and Rabbi Zoenenfeld, Beit Machaseh, 9.1.2l.1930 (CZA J113/1388).

430. Ibid.

431. Ibid.

432. Ibid.

433. Ay. Karniel, Achot ha-Tachanah, Tazkir al Chagigat Yaldei Gil ha-Maavar be-Tachanat G — Beit Yaakov (Station Nurse, Memorandum on the Passage-Age Children's Celebration at Station C — Beit Yaakov) Jerusalem, 5.9.1935 (CZA J113/1390).

434. The term "informal education" refers to guiding children and youth after school hours, in school, or after work, in a framework including social, cultural, leisure, and sports activity; Y. Meyuhas (ed.), **Thirty-Five Years of Supplementary Education**, Jerusalem, 1970, p.1.

435. The Balfour Declaration, issued on November 2, 1917, by British Foreign Minister James Arthur Balfour, promised a Jewish National Home in Palestine.

436. Miller (footnote 23).

437. A. Schmeltz, "The reduction of the population of Eretz Israel [Palestine] during the First World War, M. Eliav (ed.), **Siege and Distress: Eretz Israel During the First World Wa**r, Jerusalem, 1991 pp. 32-37.

438. Z. Greenberg, "The typhus epidemic in Palestine during the First World War," lecture at the **Annual Convention of the Israel Association for the History of Medicine and Science**, September 14, 1995.

439. Ben Gurion (footnote 7), p. 112.

440. S. Shvarts, "The development of mother and infant welfare centers in Israel 1854–1954," **Journal of the History of Medicine and Allied Sciences,** 11(2000), pp. 398-425.

441. S. Shvarts and T. M. Brown, Kupat Holim, "Dr. Isaac Max Rubinow and the American Zionist Medical Unit's Experiment to Establish Health Care Services in Palestine 1918-1923," **Bulletin of the History of Medicine**, 1998, pp. 28-46; S. Shvarts, **The Workers' Health Fund in Eretz Israel**, NY, 2002, pp. 70-92.

442. Eliezer Hoffein (1957–1991) was born in Holland, and in 1912 was one of the firsts to emigrate from Western Europe to Palestine. Until 1924, he served as the vice-director, and later the director, of the Anglo-Palestine Bank. He was the first economic expert to be a member of the Zionist Federation. During World War I, he represented the United American Aid Committee.

443. Schmaltz(footnote 437), p. 44.

444. The Guggenheimer Family Papers, Ms 1341, Jones Memorial Library, Lynchburg, VA.

445. G. Freudenberg, **Robert Owen: Educator of the People**, Tel Aviv, 1970.

446. J. Lee, **Play and Playgrounds**, New York (CZA, A419/77); D. Cardwell, "New York Tries to Think Outside the Sandbox," **The New York Times**, Jan. 1, 2007.

447. Rachel Schwartz (1898–1994), mother of Ruth Dayan and Reuma Weizmann, studied Montessori early childhood education in England and interned in leisure education. She served as the first kindergarten teacher in the Old City of Jerusalem, in a mixed kindergarten with both Arab and Jewish children.

448. "Training counselors for playgrounds and for recreational institutions," **Yediot Hadassah** [Hadassah News], July 7, 1940.

449. E. C Guggenheimer, **Planning for Parks and Recreation Needs in Urban Areas**, New York, 1969, p. 88; R. Johnson, 'Playgrounds in Practice', in T. Liftzin (ed.), **The Leisure Culture and Recreation in Palestine**, Tel Aviv, 1975, pp. 100-106.

450. Moshe Shvabe (1889–1956), born in Germany, came to Eretz Israel in 1925, and was one of the founders of supplementary education in Eretz Israel. In 1927, he founded the Scouts Legion in Jerusalem, which served as the nucleus for the first Scout youth movement in Eretz Israel. He also served for many years as head of the Pedagogic Board of the Guggenheimer–Hadassah Playgrounds.

451. Rachel Schwartz, "A Playground in Palestine," May 1933, Hadassah Archives, New York, 4/30/237.

452. According to her will, the fund was meant to remain intact, and money for the playgrounds was meant to come from the interest alone. The Hadassah administration took the execution of Guggenheimer's will upon itself and in 1930 appointed an Advisory Board to supervise the program. Minutes of the First

Meeting of the Advisory Committee of the Zion Hill Playground, Held at the Headquarters of the Hadassah Medical Organization, Jerusalem, March 11, 1928, Hadassah Archives, New York, Division 7, File 111.

453. The American trustees of the Guggenheimer Fund were Stephen Samuel Wise (1874–1949), president of the American Jewish Congress from 1939 to 1949, Judge Julian William Mack (1866–1976), president of the First Jewish Congress and president of the American Zionist Federation (1918–1921), and Irma Lindheim (1886–1976), president of Hadassah (1926–1928), and member of Kibbutz Mishmar Ha'Emek from 1933 until her death. A letter from Irma Lindheim, Mishmar Ha'Emek, to "Young Hadassah" in New York, November 8, 1939, Hadassah Archives, New York, 4/255/31; personal archives, Rachel Schwartz, CZA A419; Kibbutz Mishmar Ha'Emek archives.

454. Z. Shehory-Rubin, "Health and Recuperation in Safad: A Convalescence-Home to Save Elementary School Students from Yesod Hama'ala and Mishmar Hayarden from the Dreaded Malaria", **Dor LeDor**, 34 (2009), pp.69-71.

455. The "Machane Yehuda" neighborhood incorporated a number of slum areas — Nachalat Zion, Schunat Chaim, Sha'arei Zedek, Ohel Moshe, Zichron Yosef, and Mazkeret Yosef — all of which were densely populated by Jews of primarily Eastern (Oriental) origin —Sephardim, Persians, Kurds, and Mughrabis.

456. Ephraim Bluestone (1891–1979), physician and medical administrator, was director of Hadassah in Palestine from 1926 through 1928. Graduated in medicine in Jefferson College, Pennsylvania, specialized at Mount Sinai Hospital, and after his service in Eretz Israel, returned to direct the Montefiore Hospital in New York (now the Albert Einstein Medical Center). D. Levenson, **Montefiore: The Hospital as a Social_Instrument**, New York, 1984, pp. 146-161; S. Shvarts, "Charity or Social Right? The Controversy of the Hospitalization of Members of the Jewish Labor Federation in Palestine 1926–1928," **Israel Journal of Medical Sciences**, 32 (1996), pp. 248-253.

457. Bluestone to Bassan, June 17, 1928, Hadassah Archives, New York, 4/31/249; CZA, A419/68; "The Opening of the Guggenheimer Playground in Machane Yehuda," **Davar,** April 1929.

458. Rachel HaMeirit-Gorodisky, interview, March 7, 1994.

459. The need for playgrounds was reflected even in contemporary journalism. R. Levin, "The Situation of Infants and Mothers," **Davar,** September 1926; G. Birkham, "The Child and Society," **Ha-Isha** II, [additional issue] (1929), pp. 6-8.

460. Schwartz, interview, November 26, 1993.

461. Ibid.

462. R. Schwartz, "Towards an explanation of work methods in the playgrounds." Lecture written for the Conference of Counselors, December 1932, CZA A419/95.

463. Malka and Yosef Koriel, interview, August 10, 1994; Judge Yitzhak Banai, who played regularly at the Makor Baruch Playground, interview, March 18, 1994.

464. Children Playgrounds, **Doar Hayom** (the Daily Post, Hebrew), Jan. 22, 1934.

465. Lillian Kornfeld report, September 1925, pp.1-2, Hadassah Archives, 7/111.

466. Children Playgrounds, **Doar Hayom** (the Daily Post, Hebrew), Jan.22, 1934.

467. R. Schwartz, "Playgrounds for Children," **Ha-Isha**, 2 [additional issue] (1929), 53-55; 'Playgrounds for Children', **Doar HaYom** [newspaper], February 1934.

468. Schwartz, interview, November 26, 1993.

469. Minutes of the Second Convention of Counselors of the Guggenheimer-Hadassah Playgrounds, December 30-31, 1932 (CZA J17/432).

470. S. L. Hattis, **The Bi-National Idea in Palestine during Mandatory Times**, Haifa, 1970, pp.171-172.

471. Ibid.

472. Minutes of the Twenty-Ninth meeting of the Advisory Board of the Guggenheimer-Hadassah Playgrounds in Palestine, held at the head offices of Hadassah in Jerusalem, September 28, 1930 (CZA, J17/432).

473. Ibid.

474. R. Schwartz, "Playgrounds for Children," **Ha-Isha,** 2 [additional issue] (1929), pp. 53-55.

475. Gal (footnote 8), p.160.

476. Protokol ha-Vaadah le-Mechkar ha-Se'alah ha-Yehudit-Aravit (Protocol of the Committeee to Investiagate the Jewish Arab Question), 14 May 1940, Ben-Gurion Archives, Ben-Gurion Heritage Institute, Sede Boker, S44/149, Portfolio Hadassah, 1937–1942.

477. Rachel Schwartz, "S'kirah shel Migrachei ha-Mischakim — October–November 1929" (A Survey of the Playgrounds: October-November 1929 (CZA, A419/67).

478. The 1929 Arab Riots broke out following a protracted disagreement about the rights of Jews to pray at the Western Wall, and rumors in Arab circles that the Jews planned to take over the Temple Mount — hostility and incitement that took place against the backdrop of growing anti-Zionist militancy among the Arab community in Mandate Palestine. The primary flash points were in Jerusalem, Hebron and Safed, but attacks by armed Arab bands and murders of Jews (133 in all) took place throughout the country, and a number of Jewish communities such as Huldah and Mishmar Ha'Emek were evacuated by their Jewish inhabitants and razed by Arab marauders. The ancient Jewish community of Hebron, which had been the target of one of the worst attacks leaving 60 dead, ceased to exist after surviving Jews were evacuated by the British and forbidden to return. The 1929 Riots were a watershed event in Jewish-Arab relations.

479. Margaret G. Doniger, "Ha-iru'im ha-Trag'im" (Tragic Events) (CZA, A419/99).

480. Correspondence, Rachel Schwartz to Margaret G. Doniger, USA, dated October 5, 1930 (CZA, A419/82).

481. "Protokol Yisivat Ha-Vaadah Ha-Mezaetzet she-Hitkansah b-Yerushaliyim b-5.8.1930 k'dei la-Dun be-Atid shel Har Zion'" (Meeting of the Advisory Committee, convened in Jerusalem on August 5, 1930 to discuss the future of 'Mount Zion') (CZA, A419/73).

482. The 1936–1939 Great Arab Revolt included attacks between April 1936 and September 1939 against British rule and against Jewish settlements. In the summer of 1938 the revolt reached its peak. Police stations and trains were attacked, British civil servants were shot, and Arab gangs attacked Jewish settlements. The primary trigger behind the outbreak of the attacks was three years of large-scale Jewish immigration to Mandate Palestine (sparked by the rise of Hitler to power in Germany in 1933) that preceded its outbreak — that brought some 150,000 persons who doubled the size of the Jewish community in Eretz Israel and transformed Jewish Palestine into a powerful economic and political player. Yosef Heller, me-Me'ura'ot 1936 ad le-Milchemet Ha-Komemiyut" (From the Arab Revolt 1936 to the War of Independence") in B. Aliav (ed.), **Ha-Yishuv ha-Yehudi b-Yamei ha-Byit ha-Leumi, 1917–1948** (The Jewish Community in the Days of the National Homeland, 1917–1948), Jerusalem, 1976, pp. 61-86.

483. Minutes of Palestine Council of Hadassah, 1 September 1941.

484. Letter from Irma Lindheim to Young Hadassah, November 8, 1938, Hadassah Archives — New York, 4/31/255.

485. HaMeirit-Gorodisky, interview, March 7, 1994.

486. Nesher, interview, January 1, 1995; "Annual Report of the Hadassah Medical Organization for 1929-1930," **Yediot Hadassah**, 2 (May-June 1930), 1-6.

487. Kornfeld Report, Hadassah Archives, 7/111.

488. Schwartz, interview, November 26, 1993.

489. Ibid.

490. Rabbi Kook (1865–1935) was born in Latvia, immigrated to Eretz Israel in 1904, and served as the Chief Rabbi of Jaffa. After World

War I, he served as the Chief Rabbi of Jerusalem. In 1921, with the founding of the Chief Rabbinate, he was chosen as the Chief Ashkenazi Rabbi of Eretz Israel.

491. Schwartz, interview, November 26, 1993; M. Levin, **Balm in Gilead**, Jerusalem, 1997, p. 89. In Levin's opinion, the director of the yeshiva was furious because his granddaughter went to the playground, against his will. No additional evidence was found for this.

492. Elboim-Dror (footnote 86), p. 286.

493. Ibid.

494. Ben-Ishai's words, at the meeting of the Administrative Board of the Guggenheimer-Hadassah Playgrounds in Palestine, August 28, 1944 (CZA, J17/432). See also: B. Ben-Ishai, **Problems of Recreation in Our Society**, Jerusalem, 1962.

495. Berachiahu (footnote 186) p. 4.

496. Meeting of school doctors and nurses, June 17, 1929 (CZA J113/343).

497. Berachiahu to the Executive Board of the Hadassah Medical Organization, August 22, 1928 (CZA J113/342); S. Shvarts, Israel Health Policy and the Ringworm Case — New Findings, New Context paper presented at the **Association for Israel Studies**, 25th Annual Conference, Beer Sheva, June 2009.

498. Yaacov Yehoshua, **Jerusalem Yesterday and the Day Before** ,Jerusalem, 1977, p. 65; 166; for more on the water shortage in Jerusalem, "Bringing Water to Jerusalem by Train," **Davar**, September, 1925.

499. Koriel, interview, August 10, 1994.

500. Annual Report of Hadassah/Guggenheimer Activities for the Year 1948/49 (CZA, J17/432).

501. Yosef Meyuhas, one of the first teachers born in Palestine to work towards Arab-Jewish coexistence, was one of the central advocates of supplementary education, counselor and superintendent of

the Guggenheimer-Hadassah playgrounds, and director of the Youth Department of the Ministry of Education and Culture from 1935 through 1972; R. Schwartz, "Portrait of Yosef Meyuhas," March 18, 1977 (CZA, A419-114).

502. Y. Meyuhas, **Book of Supplementary Education**, Jerusalem, 1975, p. 217.

503. School Hygiene Department (1921).

504. Data taken from: "Mazkir Machleket Higiyena shel Batei ha-Sefer le-Shnat 1929–1930" (Memorandum — School Hygiene Department for the years 1929-30) (CZA, J113/344).

505. The School Hygiene Department treated schoolchildren and concurrently their families, too, otherwise trachoma would not have been contained. Dr. Yehudit Kozlova, a school ophthalmologist, warned that "only by curing entire families we will have really important results." Report by Dr. Kozlova to Hadassah management, 5.6.1929 (CZA J113/346); Dr. Avraham Katzenelson, member of the Secretariat for Health Matters of the National Committee, sent a report to Colonel Heron, director of the Government Health Department in which he cited that "there is no value to treatment in the schools, if there is no parallel treatment of family members of infected students." In the Government Report of Health Services 1935/6, written by Dr. Abraham Katzenelson, 5.12.1934 (CZA, J113/348).

506. Eye checkups in schools in the agricultural townships (moshavot) were carried out by a traveling doctor who underwent a special course in hygiene and sanitation and who supervised hygiene and sanitation in township schools, as well. **Yediot Hadassah**, Pamphlet 1-6, 1929, p. 26; **Ba-Galil**, 3 (1929), p. 13. On the work of Dr. Yasski as a traveling doctor (CZA J113/410). On the work of the traveling doctor in curing trachoma at various points in the country (CZA J113/415).

507. Report of Dr. Dostrovsky — Ringworm Jerusalem Schools (CZA J1113/1434).

508. Berachiahu (footnote 186), p. 5.

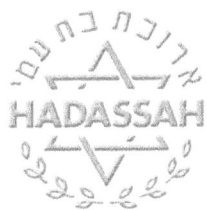

Index